Development of Oldest-Old Mortality, 1950-1990:
Evidence from 28 Developed Countries

MONOGRAPHS ON POPULATION AGING

General Editors
Bernard Jeune and James W. Vaupel

Development of Oldest-Old Mortality, 1950-1990:
Evidence from 28 Developed Countries
Väinö Kannisto

Aging Research Unit
Centre for Health and Social Policy
Odense University Medical School

Development of oldest-old mortality, 1950-1990: Evidence from 28 developed countries

Väinö Kannisto

Monographs on Population Aging, 1.

Odense University Press

Development of oldest-old mortality, 1950-1990:
Evidence from 28 Developed Countries
© Väinö Kannisto and Odense University Press, 1994
Printed by Special-Trykkeriet Viborg a-s
Cover design by Ulla Poulsen Precht
Cover illustration: Jens Bohr's color woodcut "Salmonsen at the furthest Sea"
ISBN 87 7838 015 4
ISSN 0909-119 X

Contents

Preface 9

Acknowledgements 11

I. The Data 13
    1. Data on mortality of the oldest-old 13
    2. Data quality 14
    3. Cohort survival histories 16
    4. Current survivors 18
    5. What does the database represent? 19

II. Findings 21
    6. Growing numbers of old people 21
    7. Proportion of the oldest-old in total population 23
    8. Mortality of the oldest-old since 1950 27
    9. Onset of sustained mortality decline 41
    10. Age pattern of mortality decline 47
    11. The case of centenarians 51
    12. Period or cohort effect? 55
    13. Sex ratio and sex differential of mortality 59
    14. Effect of differential mortality on population sex ratio .. 63
    15. Conclusion 66

Sources 68

References 69

Annex Tables 70
by Väinö Kannisto, Jens Lauritsen, Kirill Andreev

List of Tables and Figures

Tables

1. Kannisto-Thatcher Oldest-Old Database 12
2. Growth of the oldest-old population from 1950 to 1990 22
3. Growth factor of the oldest-old population from 1950 to 1990,
   by country 23
4. Proportion of the oldest-old in total population, 1960 and 1990,
   by country 24
5. Proportion of centenarians in total population, 1960 and 1990,
   by country 26
6. Age-standardized death rates at ages 80 - 99 in 1955-59 and
   1985-89, by country. Total and annual decline 31
7. Age-standardized death rates at 80 - 99 years in groups of
   countries 32
8. Ranking of countries according to mortality at ages 80 - 99
   in 1955-59 and 1985-89. Both sexes 36
9. Decline of mortality at ages 80 - 99 from 1955-59 to 1985-89 39
10. Onset of sustained decline in old-age mortality 42
11. Annual decline of mortality at ages 80-99. Calculated from the
    mean for the last 5 years relatively to the mean for
    the preceding 5 years 44
12. Decline of mortality by age and sex from 1955-59 to 1985-89,
    percent 49
13. Probability of dying at ages 100 and over, 1980-1990 52
14. Percent change in age-specific death rate from given 5-year
    period to the next. Selected countries 58
15. Sex ratios of mortality at ages 80 - 99 years, by country 61

Figures

1. Lexis diagram with age (x), year (y) and cohort (z) 17
2a. Death rates at ages 80 - 99 years. Males 28
2b. Death rates at ages 80 - 99 years. Females 29
3. Death rates at ages 80 - 99 in 1955-59 and 1985-89.
   Both sexes 37
4. Relative decline of mortality at ages 80 - 99 from 1955-59
   to 1985-89 40
5. Relative change of mortality by age and sex from 1955-59
   to 1985-89. Selected countries 46
6. Deaths per 1000 population age 100 and over in 13 countries
   of Western Europe 53
7. Probability of dying at ages 100 and over 54
8. Percent change in age-specific death rate. Selected countries 56
9. Sex ratio of mortality by age 62
10. Sex differential of mortality per 1000 population by age 64
11. Sex ratio of population aged 80 and over 65

Annex tables

1. Persons and deaths in 1950-1990 in the Kannisto-Thatcher Oldest-Old Database 71
2. Age-standardized death rates at ages 80 - 99 in 1950-1990 28 countries 72
3. Age-standardized death rates at ages 80 - 99 by 5-year periods in 1950-1989. 28 countries 80
4. Age-standardized death rates at ages 80 - 99 in 1950-1990 Selected groups of countries 84
5. Age-standardized death rates at ages 80-99. Average of last five annual rates. Male/Female 86
6. Mortality of the elderly in 1955-59 and 1985-89 by age and sex. Selected countries 94
7. Death rates by age and sex in 1950-1989. Groups of countries. 97
8. Deaths per 1000 population aged 100 and over in 1950-1989 in Western Europe 101
9. Probability of dying at ages 100 and over by decade 102
10. Sex ratio of mortality at ages 80 - 99, by country 104
11. Sex ratio of mortality by age by groups of countries 106
12. Standard population: Sweden, both sexes, 1950-1989 108

Preface

Until recently octogenarians were unusual and centenarians rare. Today, close to half of female deaths and a third of male deaths in developed countries occur among those above age 80, and 100,000 or more centenarians may celebrate the turn of the century. Data bases have not kept up with this new demography: researchers are thwarted by the lack of more extensive, more reliable data on mortality and morbidity at advanced ages. The Odense Archive of Population Data on Aging was established in 1992 at Odense University Medical School to help meet the pressing need.

This monograph by Väinö Kannisto, former United Nations advisor on demographic and social statistics, is the first of a series that will analyze data contained in the Odense Archive of Population Data on Aging. It is fitting that Kannisto is the author of the first monograph because the core set of data in the archive was assembled, tested for quality, and converted into cohort mortality histories by him. These data, which pertain to death counts and population counts by year of age, year of birth, and current year over the last four decades or so in some thirty countries, permit the estimation of death rates after age 80. Also included in the data base and analyzed in this report are comparable materials on England and Wales, made available by A. Roger Thatcher, former Director of the Office of Population Censuses and Surveys and Registrar-General of England and Wales. Kannisto and Thatcher used the same extinct-cohort method to estimate population counts from death counts.

Stimulus for the establishment of the Kannisto-Thatcher Oldest-Old Database was provided by Peter Laslett, Advisory Director of Cambridge Group for the History of Population and Social Structure, who invited Kannisto, Thatcher and me to join him in an ongoing Cambridge-based project on Maximal Length of Life. With research funding provided by the U.S. National Institute on Aging and the Danish Research Councils, the Kannisto and Thatcher data bases were computerized at the Aging Research Unit of the Centre for Health and Social Policy at Odense University Medical School. In addition to Kannisto, Thatcher, and myself, Jens Lauritsen, Kirill Andreev, and Zeng Xuhui played major roles in this task. Lauritsen and Andreev are co-authors, with Kannisto, of the data annex of this monograph.

The Kannisto-Thatcher Oldest-Old Database and several other data bases relevant to population studies of aging comprise the Odense Archive of Population Data on Aging. The other data bases include the following.

Hans Lundström has completed a data base of highly reliable death counts and populations counts for Sweden by single year of time since 1865 for ages 50 and older.

Kirill Andreev and Axel Skytthe, with considerable help from Ulla Larsen and Jens Lauritsen, have created a similar data base for Denmark, with ages from birth onwards and starting in 1830.

James R. Carey, Professor at the University of California at Davis, and James W. Curtsinger, Professor at the University of Minnesota, have contributed their data on the lifespans of fruitflies. Their experiments, by far the largest concerning the mortality of any non-human species, permit estimation of death rates at advanced ages for Medflies, Mexican fruit flies and *Drosophila*.

Under the leadership of Professors Mogens Hauge and Bent Harvald, the Danish Twin Registry was established at Odense University Medical School. Data on lifespans of twins born in Denmark between 1870 and 1930 have been included in the Odense Archive of Population Data on Aging. These data are uniquely valuable for genetic studies of aging: no other twin registry traces, from childhood on, twins born in the 19th century.

Additional data are being assembled and added to the Archive. The Kannisto-Thatcher, Lundström and Danish data bases on human mortality are being regularly updated and, for some countries, extended further back in time and to younger ages. Additional fruit fly data are being collected. Data, both from historical and archaeological sources, are being gathered pertaining to changes in the length of human lifespans from the Mesolithic to modern times. Information about the health, morbidity, and disability of elderly Danish twins and of Danish centenarians will be provided by research projects now underway.

The Kannisto-Thatcher Oldest-Old Database and the larger Odense Archive of Population Data on Aging are managed by the Aging Research Unit of the Centre for Health and Social Policy at the Odense University Medical School. Computerized data from the Archive are available through the Danish Data Archives, a division of the Danish national library system, located in Odense. Researchers interested in using data from the Archive should write to me at the Aging Research Unit, Odense University Medical School, Winsloewparken 17, 5000 Odense, Denmark.

Professor James W. Vaupel

Acknowledgements

A reliable, though still incomplete description of the human life span is possible today only thanks to the foresight and careful management by government statisticians in various countries beginning with the foundation of Tabell-verket in Stockholm in 1749. Guardians of this tradition of public statistics, today's responsible officials in national statistical agencies, too numerous to be listed here, have generously contributed their time and counsel to the assembly of information for our database.

The author is grateful to James W. Vaupel for having made possible the computerization of the data and the publication of this report, to A.R. Thatcher for joining his data on England and Wales to the database and to both for many stimulating discussions about the subject. Thanks are also due to Peter Laslett for furthering the study of the maximal length of life by several meetings in Cambridge. The author thanks Jens Lauritsen, Zeng Xuhui and Kirill Andreev for their assiduous work in computerizing the very large volume of data. In particular, Lauritsen has been instrumental in organizing the database under the supervision of Vaupel, and Andreev in producing the final tables and figures of this report. The author also thanks Lis Bluhme and Lise Stark for typing the text, and Bernard Jeune for arrangements with the editor.

Comments on the present report should be addressed to me at Campo Grande 1-6-D, 1700 Lisbon, Portugal.

Väinö Kannisto

Table 1.   KANNISTO-THATCHER OLDEST-OLD DATABASE

Country or area	Period	Age/year of birth[1]	Ages covered[2]	Sub-categories
Australia	1965-90	A	80+	
Austria	1947-91	A	80+	
Belgium	1950-91	A/Y	80+	
Canada	1950-88	A	80-99	
Chile	1980-88	A	80-104	
Czechoslovakia	1950-90	A/Y	80-100	
Denmark	1924-90	A/Y	80+	
England & Wales	1911-90	A	80+	
Estonia	1950-91	A	80-99	
Finland	1878-1990	A/Y	80+	
France	1950-91	A/Y	80+	
Germany, East	1954-91	A	80-99	
Germany, West	1951-91	A/Y	80+	
Hungary	1950-90	A/Y	80-99	
Iceland	1961-90	A/Y	80+	
Ireland	1950-89	A	80+	
Italy	1952-89	A/Y	80+	
Japan	1950-91	A/Y	80+	
Latvia	1950-90	A	80-99	
Luxemburg	1953-89	A	80-99	
Netherlands	1960-91	A/Y	80+	
New Zealand	1950-90	A	80+	non-Maori/Maori
Norway	1911-90	A/Y	80+	
Poland	1971-90	A/Y	80-99	
Portugal	1940-90	A	80+	
Scotland	1950-91	A	80-99	
Singapore	1982-91	A	80+	Chinese
Spain	1950-86	A/Y	80+	
Sweden	1920-90	A/Y	80+	
Switzerland	1950-91	A/Y	80+	
United States	1960-88	A	85+	white/others

[1]   A   = data classified by age alone
      A/Y = data cross-classified by age and year of birth

[2]   80+   = data by single years without upper age limit
      80-99 = data by single years from 80 to 99, then 100+

Data were assembled and prepared by V. Kannisto, except for England and Wales which were similarly prepared by A.R. Thatcher.

I. The Data

1. Data on the mortality of the oldest-old

The compilation of the data which have been used for the present report and, it is hoped, will be used for many studies to follow, began as a hobby in statistical libraries in Lisbon, Helsinki and Geneva, originally to satisfy the curiosity as to what is happening at the top of the age pyramid. It soon became clear that for a comprehensive view direct assistance of national statistical offices was necessary. In international conferences and by correspondence the author therefore contacted, beginning in 1987, responsible officials of 48 countries most likely to have data on deaths at old age, sufficiently reliable and detailed for application of the method of extinct generations of Paul Vincent which from the beginning was considered to be the method of choice for the purpose.

Positive response was received from 42 countries and ultimately material from 30 among them were found suitable for due and uniform treatment and were arranged into cohort mortality histories. A.R. Thatcher had undertaken to do the same for England and Wales and so contributed this indispensable element to the international picture. Following an offer by James W. Vaupel, the data for all 31 countries were computerized at the University of Odense to form the *Kannisto-Thatcher Oldest-Old Database* within the *Odense Archive of Population Data on Aging*.

The intention has been to assemble mortality statistics on old persons from all countries which process them by sex and single years of age, preferably combined with the year of birth and without any upper limit or at least up to age 99. The sources include official publications as well as unpublished materials made available by national statistical agencies, in some cases specially tabulated at request.

The stored data begin at age 80 and start for most countries with the year 1950. Some series, however, begin at a later date while some others reach back to last century. The latest year on record varies by country but is at this time in most cases 1990 or 1991.

The geographic coverage of countries fulfilling the data requirements is nearly complete but efforts will continue to expand it and to encourage more countries to produce comparable data. The contents of the database as of this writing are summed up in Table 1.

2. Data quality

The data on deaths have been subjected to a number of tests on their plausibility and internal consistency. While age heaping is easily observed in age-specific death rates, evidence of age overstatement can be detected by examining age distributions of deaths. Measurement of the slope of mortality is also apt to reveal dubious patterns caused by overstatement of age. As this error is almost invariably greater among old men than women, it usually leads to an abnormal sex ratio. Countries with data of proven high quality provide a set of indicators against which less certain data can be compared. At the opposite end, indicators found in notoriously unreliable data show the direction and magnitude of alarm signals. Another diagnostic tool are time series of data quality indicators which often reveal improvement over time towards more plausible levels. As a whole the data quality indicators for the 30-odd countries present a consistent and logical picture with a range of values in which it is possible to discern various degrees of reliability with some assurance when due regard is paid to the degree of aging and the general level of mortality in the country in question. A report on quality assessment of the Kannisto-Thatcher database will be published in a forthcoming volume in this series.

On the basis of these findings the data have been classified into the following four quality categories.

A. Good quality

Austria	Iceland
Belgium	Italy
Czechoslovakia	Japan
Denmark	Luxemburg
England and Wales[1]	Netherlands
Finland	Norway
France	Scotland[1]
Germany, East[2]	Sweden
Germany, West[2]	Switzerland
Hungary	

---

[1] England and Wales on one hand and Scotland on the other will be treated as separate countries because their vital statistics are prepared and published separately.

[2] The two parts of Germany before reunification will be called East and West Germany, as this may be more convenient than acronyms because different readers have been used to acronyms based on different languages.

Although quality differences can be noted within this group of 19, it has not been found easy nor important to divide it into sub-groups. For the following five countries the data go in single years to age 99 only: Czechoslovakia, Germany (East), Hungary, Luxemburg, Scotland. The three first-mentioned among them form an analytically very useful group of the former East bloc. The data for the remaining 14 countries will be frequently used as the source of the most reliable information available on the human life span. It should be noted, however, that the Italian data for 1950s and the early Japanese data on centenarians were not fully reliable and that pre-1960 data on Iceland and the Netherlands are missing.

B. Acceptable quality

> Australia
> New Zealand, non-Maori[3]
> Portugal
> Singapore, Chinese[4]

The Australian data show an apparent increase in mortality at ages 100-104 which is probably due to data improvement while it is not known whether this has already run its course. The New Zealand data are affected by uncertain age information on South Pacific immigrants who are classified as non-Maoris. Both countries show an unusually high proportion of deaths over age 100 which may or may not be true. The quality indicators for Portugal show notable improvement over time resulting in approximately correct data for the last two decades except at ages over 105. The series for Singapore is as yet too short for conclusive evaluation.

C. Conditionally acceptable quality

> Estonia
> Ireland
> Latvia
> Poland
> Spain

---

[3] Data for New Zealand, unless otherwise stated, refer to the non-Maori population only. The Maori population is small and the data for it unreliable.
[4] Data for Singapore refer to the Chinese population only. Data for other ethnic groups are available but are too small to be significant.

These data give probably a roughly correct description of the mortality trend though at a level artificially lowered by age overstatement. The Estonian data are considerably better than those for Latvia and Poland.

D. Weak quality

>Canada
>Chile
>New Zealand, Maori
>United States

Used with due caution, these data may give approximate information on the size and development of the old age population below age 90 or 100 but estimation of mortality by the method applied in this report would be too uncertain. The data on Chile, New Zealand Maoris and United States non-whites are clearly the least reliable.

3. Cohort survival histories

The database has been constructed from data on deaths arranged into cohort survival histories. This procedure can be illustrated with a Lexis diagram (Figure 1) where age is on the vertical and time on the horizontal scale. Each person can be understood to advance diagonally in the up-and-right direction, crossing horizontal lines (birthdays) and vertical New Year days but remaining in his/her cohort (determined by the year of birth) until his/her individual line ends in death.

The vital statistics annually published by national offices customarily give the number of deaths in year y at each age x (age last birthday): square ABCD in the diagram. Many countries - fortunately for our purpose - also divide the deaths according to the year of birth, thus giving them separately for the triangles ABD and BCD. This information allows the construction of the mortality history of a cohort from deaths in successive triangles (ABD, ADE, DEF, EFG etc.) and it has been available for Belgium, Czechoslovakia, Denmark, Finland, France, Germany (West), Hungary, Iceland, Italy, Japan, Netherlands, Norway (until 1976), Poland, Spain, Sweden and Switzerland.

For countries which do not indicate the year of birth, the deaths in a Lexis square have been split into the two triangles at an arbitrary ratio. Data from countries with full information show that the ratio at old ages is, on the average, close to an even 50/50 split unless an unusual event has occurred or the numbers are small. For some countries in the database the split was made at a ratio observed in a neighbouring country but in most cases the 50/50 ratio was used. This can be considered adequate for period analysis but not for cohort analysis because it ignores the often unequal size of adjacent cohorts which may reflect short-term fluctuations in birth rate in the past.

VINCENT concluded (1951) that when a cohort has died out, its size in any past year and age can be obtained by summing up the deaths beginning with the oldest. International migration is at old age small enough to be ignored. Subsequently his "method of extinct generations" has been used by many researchers to study mortality at ages 80 or 85 years and higher, and the accuracy of the method at these ages has been generally recognized. This age limitation may be more strict than what is necessary. This author demonstrated (1990) by simulation that it can be successfully applied even to province data from age 65 or 55.

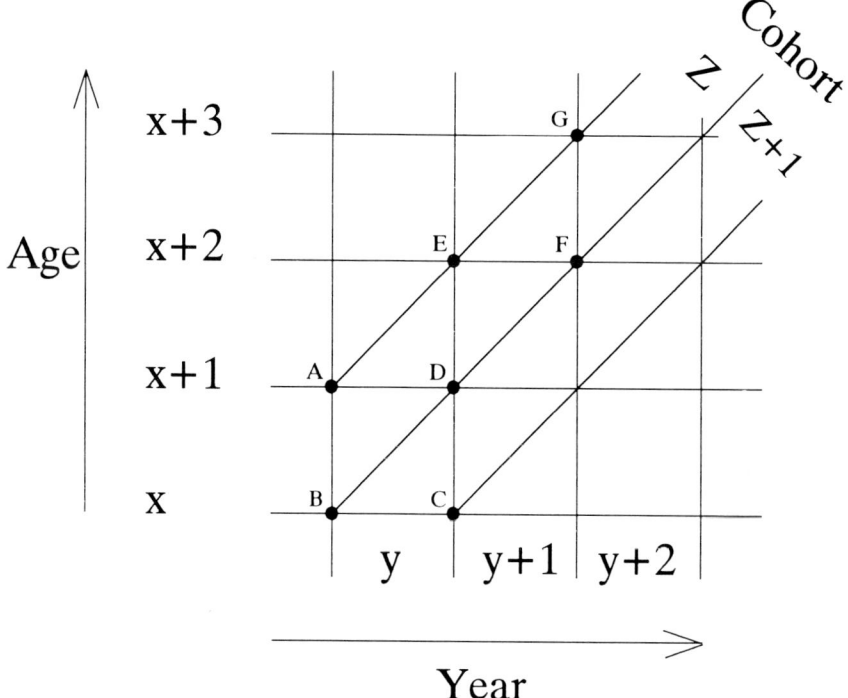

Figure 1. Lexis diagram with age (x), year (y) and cohort (z).

We have applied this method in the database even for countries in which highly accurate population registers produce data on population by age and sex; in these cases the two sets of exposed-to-risk are almost identical and though the register figure may be more correct, the cumulated figure is more practical because of its consistency with data on deaths.

For cohorts which are not yet extinct, the number of current survivors has to be determined (see Chapter 4) before the deaths are summed up.

The decision to build the database on cohort histories was not motivated by a belief that cohort is the decisive or even an important factor in mortality. The main reason was that probabilities of death can be calculated most accurately when a closed group of persons is followed from one exact age to the next, and accuracy becomes increasingly important when the numbers are small as they are at the oldest ages. The cohort structure is also practical in the management and periodic updating of the files. The Odense database can be used equally well to study period mortality as cohort mortality - the latter, however, accurately only for the 16 countries listed above which have provided data by year of birth.

The present study deals with time series and therefore does not use probabilities of death (q_x) but central death rates (m_x) as is customary in studies of age-specific mortality over time.

4. Current survivors

With current survivors we understand here the persons who were alive at the date when the information on deaths ends. This is always a year-end and therefore each year of age will correspond to one cohort.

The number of survivors has been determined on the basis of more or less independent sources such as permanent population registers, population censuses, official estimates and our own estimates derived from the deaths under the assumption that recent age-specific survival ratios in two or more successive cohorts have been identical or have changed linearly. The assumption of an identical survival ratio at a given age in successive cohorts was already used by DEPOID (1973). A report on the procedures as used in the Kannisto-Thatcher database is under preparation.

The experience with the assessment of the sources has been that good population registers produce the best and indeed very reliable population data up to the highest ages. However, countries which do not have them form the majority of the database and include all the larger ones. The official population data for these, while reliable at most ages, are often unreliable and even implausible at ages approaching or exceeding 100 years. Reflecting this uncertainty they are given by many statistical offices only in a lump sum such as "90 and over". When the lump sum has been close to our "own estimate", we have accepted it and prorated it to individual ages according to the latter. If the two have been wide apart, we have accepted our own estimate on the grounds that, though not exact, it is consistent with the information on deaths and generally plausible. With younger ages our own estimates become increasingly uncertain while the official estimates tend to become more reliable. Therefore, as a rule, at a given age we have switched to the official figure. Quite often the switch has been made easy by the fact that the two series have come very close or even identical at some age around 95 or 90 years.

5. What does the database represent?

If a low-mortality population is defined by life expectancy at birth of 75 years or more, about 780 million people, or 15 percent of the world population, enjoy low mortality. Of these, 755 million live in countries included in the database. However, the data for 277 million among them (in Canada and the United States) present considerable inaccuracies in age information, leaving 478 million in 19 low-mortality countries with essentially reliable data. The database includes further nine countries with a combined population of 102 million for which the information is judged good or acceptable; in them the life expectancy varies from 70 to 74 years. Thus the fully utilizable information covers 28 countries with a total population of 580 million in 1990, all with a life expectancy of at least 70 years.

The database may therefore be considered representative of today's low-mortality nations which it depicts in their appreciable variety and not as a uniform population. In fact, it will be seen that it has not been possible to go very far even in forming groups of countries with distinct scenarios. The spearhead of longevity is no doubt represented in the data and so are cases of various degrees of delay and stagnation in mortality reduction.

There is uncertainty as to the level of old age mortality in Canada and the U.S. but we have seen no valid evidence to assume that it in either of them falls outside the range observed in the 28 countries here described.

The population in the group of 28 is relatively aged so that while it makes up only 11 percent of the world's inhabitants, it comprises an estimated 30 percent of the 80-and-over and probably more than 40 percent of the world's centenarians.

To conclude this chapter with a word about the volume of data, the evidence from the 28 countries is based for the 1950-89 period on 68 million persons aged 80 and over of whom 51 million had died and 17 million were alive on 1st January, 1990.

The bulk of this evidence was provided by the 19 countries with good quality data, namely 58.9 million persons followed through 336 million years of exposure-to-risk resulting in 44.5 million deaths. The data are given by country in Annex Table 1.

II. Findings

6. *Growing numbers of old people*

During the early stages of the mortality transition the death rates did not change very much at old age. Although declining tendencies were observed in some countries already in the nineteenth and early twentieth century, there were also periods of stagnation and increase. For old persons, the remaining expectation of life did not increase substantially and their numbers grew only slowly as more people survived to retirement age.

In the last two or three decades a new factor has come into play: an unprecedented decline in age-specific mortality of the oldest-old themselves which has caused the life expectancy at ages 80, 90, even 100, to increase. Even though the reductions in mortality have at these ages usually been smaller than below age 80, the cumulative effect of the change has been to increase the numbers of the very oldest most rapidly in relative terms. In low-mortality countries the oldest-old are now the most rapidly growing segment of the population and, among them, it is the number of centenarians that is growing at the fastest pace.

Aggregated data for twelve countries with the most accurate information in Table 2 show that during the last 40 years the number of octogenarians has grown 4-fold, that of nonagenarians 8-fold and that of centenarians more than 20-fold. At each age the growth has been larger among females than males and the sex ratio has become increasingly lopsided, women outnumbering men 2:1 and among centenarians 5:1.

If we look at the oldest-old as a single group, more countries can be brought into comparison because uncertainty about centenarians in them hardly affects the figures. Table 3 gives the 40-year growth factor in 26 countries. In most of them the growth factor falls into the narrow range between 2.5 and 3.5. As the data for Canada and Ireland are not very trustworthy, this leaves only three countries clearly outside the range: Japan in a class of its own with an explosive 8-fold increase, trailed in some distance by Finland and Switzerland. All three are countries where the older age groups were until recently quite small. At the opposite end we find such countries of traditionally great longevity as Iceland, the Netherlands and Norway where, not surprisingly, the additional growth in numbers has been more moderate in relative terms. East Germany ranks low because of slow progress in survival.

The number of women, already larger than that of men to begin with, has continued to grow at a faster speed. There are only three exceptions to this: Japan which presents characteristics of its own, and Spain and Portugal where the 1950 data were not very reliable.

The momentum of change makes it likely that the old age populations in low-mortality countries will continue to grow rapidly and even at increasing speed.

Table 2. GROWTH OF THE OLDEST-OLD POPULATION FROM 1950 TO 1990. Pooled data for 12 countries[1]

Age	Sex	Population on 1 January		Growth factor
		1950	1990	
80-89	Males	1 164 309	3 663 310	3.1
	Females	1 850 361	7 654 426	4.1
	Total	3 014 670	11 317 736	3.8
90-99	Males	49 577	297 407	6.0
	Females	113 855	988 886	8.7
	Total	163 432	1 286 293	7.9
100+	Males	173	2 945	17.0
	Females	636	14 890	23.4
	Total	809	17 835	22.0
Total	Males	1 214 059	3 963 662	3.3
	Females	1 964 852	8 658 202	4.4
	Total	3 178 911	12 621 864	4.0

[1] Austria, Belgium, Denmark, England & Wales, Finland, France, Germany (West), Italy, Japan, Norway, Sweden and Switzerland.

Table 3. GROWTH FACTOR OF THE OLDEST-OLD POPULATION FROM 1950 TO 1990

Country or area	Total	Males	Females
Japan	7.90	8.26	7.72
Finland	4.85	4.20	5.14
Switzerland	4.65	3.94	5.09
Canada	3.91	2.93	4.72
Denmark	3.65	2.71	4.39
Germany, West	3.53	2.33	4.43
Austria	3.47	2.53	4.11
Sweden	3.36	2.70	3.87
New Zealand	3.36	2.58	3.97
Italy	3.25	2.44	3.89
Hungary	3.22	2.37	3.87
Luxemburg	3.20	2.13	4.03
France	3.19	2.83	3.37
Spain	3.17	3.22	3.14
Czechoslovakia	3.07	2.30	3.60
Belgium	2.90	2.17	3.39
Portugal	2.89	3.10	2.79
England & Wales	2.88	2.41	3.13
Estonia	2.83	2.39	3.00
Latvia	2.83	2.53	2.96
Norway	2.82	2.32	3.17
Netherlands	2.75	1.86	3.49
Scotland	2.51	1.94	2.83
Iceland	2.50	2.48	2.50
Germany, East	2.37	1.65	2.86
Ireland	1.77	1.38	2.10

7. *Proportion of the oldest-old in total population*

Persons aged 80 years and over do not yet form a large part of the total population in any country but considering the support and care they need, they are a significant factor in many societies.

The number and proportion of the oldest-old is shown in Table 4 for 30 countries. Though the numbers are often not precise, the proportion in total population can be

Table 4. PROPORTION OF THE OLDEST-OLD IN TOTAL POPULATION, 1960 AND 1990

Country	1.1.1960			1.1.1990		
	Population '000	Aged 80+	%	Population '000	Aged 80+	%
Australia	...	...	...	17 086	362 115	2.12
Austria	7 081	121 225	1.71	7 791	277 808	3.57
Belgium	9 153	169 173	1.85	9 845	347 150	3.53
Canada	17 814	224 085	1.26	26 603	589 457	2.22
Chile	...	...	...	13 173	116 070	0.88
Czechoslovakia	13 654	149 761	1.10	15 661	353 829	2.26
Denmark	4 581	73 409	1.60	5 140	188 483	3.67
England & Wales	45 862	895 104	1.95	50 950	1 863 372	3.66
Estonia	1 197	19 227	1.61	1 571	40 387	2.57
Finland	4 429	40 594	0.92	4 986	138 281	2.77
France	45 542	909 205	2.00	56 735	2 084 462	3.67
Germany, East	17 241	314 798	1.83	16 247	541 034	3.33
Germany, West	53 373	836 638	1.57	63 232	2 394 224	3.79
Hungary	9 999	108 238	1.08	10 365	259 632	2.50
Iceland	176	2 526	1.44	255	6 321	2.48
Ireland	...	...	...	3 503	77 235	2.20
Italy	49 361	777 347	1.57	57 662	1 745 513	3.03
Japan	93 200	639 409	0.69	123 537	2 823 387	2.29
Latvia	2 093	37 293	1.78	2 683	72 125	2.69
Luxemburg	314	4 683	1.49	381	11 338	2.98
Netherlands	11 480	155 340	1.35	14 952	427 964	2.86
New Zealand	2 372	35 512	1.50	3 347	72 575	2.17
Norway	3 586	70 138	1.96	4 241	156 279	3.68
Poland	...	...	...	38 180	733 676	1.92
Portugal	8 921	108 271	1.21	9 868	249 595	2.53
Scotland	5 254	84 939	1.62	4 970	166 308	3.35
Singapore	...	...	...	2 705	23 430	0.87
Spain	30 128	367 675	1.22	38 959	960 691	2.47
Sweden	7 480	137 960	1.84	8 559	359 044	4.19
Switzerland	5 351	80 707	1.51	6 712	243 975	3.63
25 countries	449 642	6 363 257	1.42	545 252	16 373 234	3.00
30 countries	...	...	...	619 899	17 685 760	2.85

considered a reasonable approximation even for countries with less reliable information. The highest proportion - 4.2 percent - is recorded in Sweden while other Scandinavian and Central European countries generally have ratios exceeding 3.5 percent as a result of early demographic transition combined with low mortality of the elderly. Low proportions are found in non-European countries which still have relatively young populations, as well as in some Eastern European countries of relatively high mortality.

In the 25 countries for which we have comparable data for 1960 and 1990, the proportion oldest-old more than doubled from 1.4 to 3.0 percent.

When the oldest-old are joined with other elderly, they form a proportion 5 to 7 times as large as they do alone. Such a segment possesses considerable political power in the countries of the database all of which are now democracies.

The impact of the on-going aging process is perhaps best measured as the increase in the proportion oldest-old in terms of percentage points rather than as relative increase which would be less meaningful in countries starting at a low base figure. Between 1960 and 1990 the proportion of oldest-old grew by the following percentage points in the total population:

Country	Value	Country	Value
Sweden	2.35	Germany, East	1.50
Germany, West	2.22	Luxemburg	1.49
Switzerland	2.12	Italy	1.46
Denmark	2.07	Hungary	1.42
Austria	1.86	Portugal	1.32
Finland	1.85	Spain	1.25
Scotland	1.73	Czechoslovakia	1.16
Norway	1.72	Iceland	1.04
England & Wales	1.71	Canada	0.96
Belgium	1.68	Estonia	0.96
France	1.67	Latvia	0.91
Japan	1.60	New Zealand	0.67
Netherlands	1.51		

The nine countries with the largest increase, more than 1.7, form a contiguous area in Central and Northern Europe. Slightly smaller increases are recorded in countries immediately to the West - Benelux and France - and still smaller ones in Southern and Eastern Europe. In these latter areas the impact of extreme aging is therefore more moderate for the time being, and the same applies to Japan.

The proportion of centenarians is expressed in Table 5 per million population. The highest ratios, around 60-70 per million, are found in countries in which the demographic transition took place early and old age mortality has been low for some time. In Japan the ratio is still as low as 25 because the development there is of a recent origin.

The extremely rapid build-up of the centenarian population is evident in its growth from 5.3 to 45.1 per million in only 30 years in the aggregate with the most precise data.

Table 5.   PROPORTION OF CENTENARIANS IN TOTAL POPULATION, 1960 AND 1990.

Country	1.1.1960		1.1.1990	
	Number	Per million	Number	Per million
Austria	25	3.5	232	29.8
Belgium	...	...	474	48.1
Denmark	19	4.1	323	62.8
England & Wales	531	11.6	3890	76.3
Estonia	...	...	42	26.7
Finland	11	2.5	141	28.3
France	371	8.1	3853	67.9
Germany, West	119	2.2	2528	40.0
Iceland	3	17.0	17	66.7
Ireland	...	...	87	24.8
Italy	265	5.4	2047	35.5
Japan	155	1.7	3126	25.3
Netherlands	62	5.4	818	54.7
New Zealand	18	7.6	198	59.2
Norway	73	20.4	300	70.7
Portugal	...	...	268	27.2
Singapore	...	...	41	15.2
Sweden	72	9.6	583	68.1
Switzerland	29	5.4	338	50.4
14 countries	1753	5.3	18 394	45.1
19 countries	...	...	19 306	44.3

The centenarians are everywhere still a quite small fraction of the population, less than one in 10,000 in all reliably documented countries but this limit is expected to be passed very soon on a broad front.

8. *Mortality of the oldest-old since 1950*

This chapter attempts to describe the present levels of oldest-old mortality in low-mortality countries and the changes that have taken place in them during the post-war period. Relying only on data of good or acceptable quality, the description is necessarily centred on Europe. From other continents prime evidence is available on Japan and more tentative results for Australia, New Zealand and Singapore.

In this study mortality is measured by central death rates (m_x) which have been calculated for 5-year age groups and individual calendar years. Age-adjusted death rates for ages 80-99 have been used as an overall indicator of oldest-old mortality[1].

From this indicator, ages of 100 years and over were left out because the necessary data were lacking for eight countries and unreliable for a few others; the effect of this age limitation is negligible because there are more than a thousand 80-99-year-old per each centenarian. For greater stability, moving averages and 5-year period rates are also used. Data for both sexes combined were calculated using weights: 1 for males, 2 for females. The decline of mortality is expressed as percentage decline of the age-adjusted rate in the 30-year period from 1955-59 to 1985-89 and it is also shown per annum. The "present" situation in the text refers to the last-mentioned period.

The post-war development in old age mortality is shown in Annex Table 2 in the form of annual age-adjusted death rates at ages 80-99 for all 28 countries for which we have at least conditionally acceptable data. Annex Table 3 gives the same for 5-year periods and Annex Table 4 for selected aggregates of countries.

The time series for 12 countries, selected for their accuracy and characteristic features, and twice smoothed with 3-year moving averages, are shown in Figures 2a and 2b in colour.

---

[1] The weights, calculated according to the Swedish population in the database in 1950-89, were the following: 80-84: 0.6360; 85-89: 0.2743; 90-94: 0.0774; 95-99: 0.0123. For the detailed standard population, see Annex Table 12.
Rates for both sexes combined have been calculated using weights 1/3 for males and 2/3 for females based on the fact that in the combined population aged 80 and over in the 19 countries with good quality data the percentage of males was 38.8 in 1950 and 31.2 in 1990. It is practical to have constant weights for all periods, countries and ages.

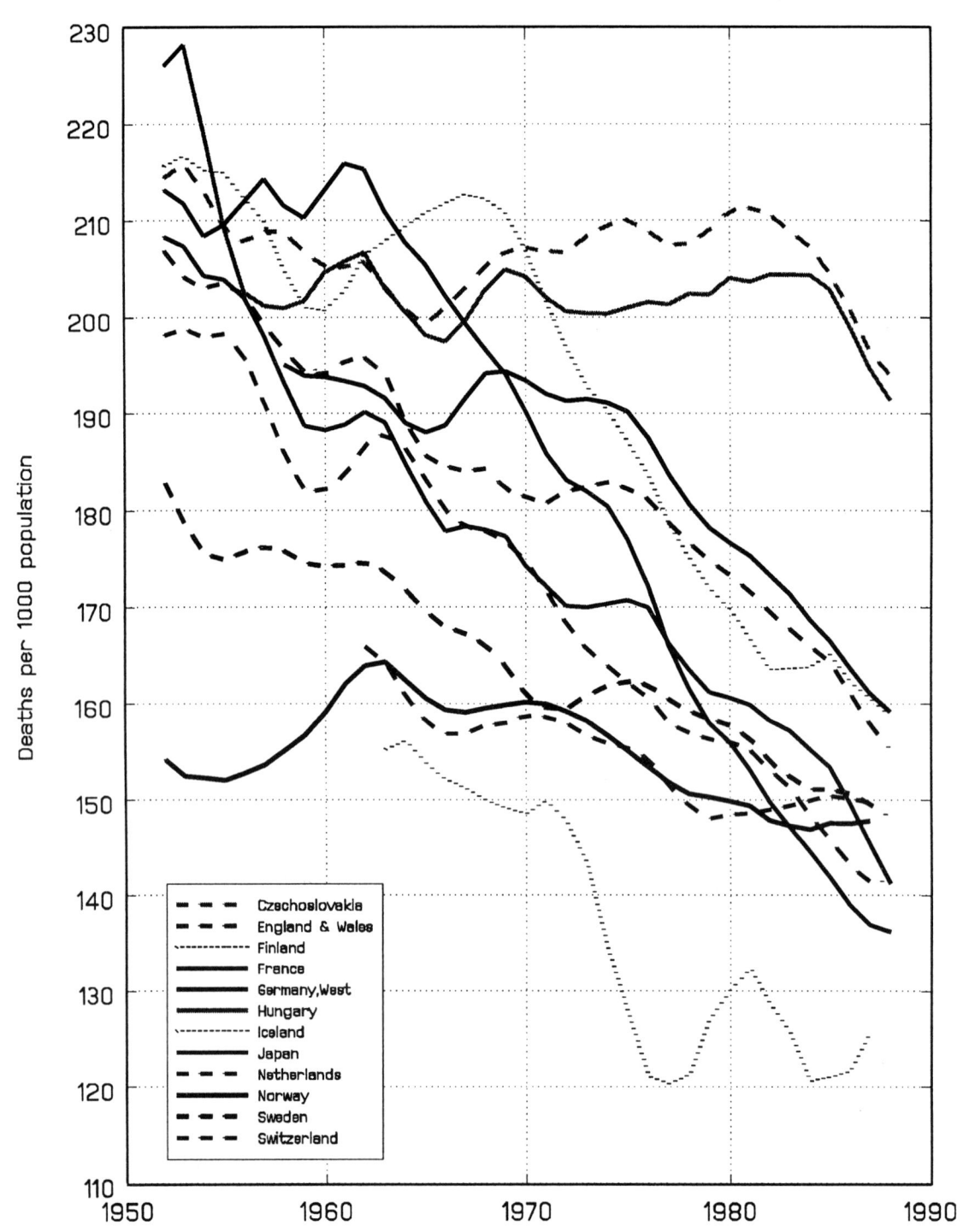

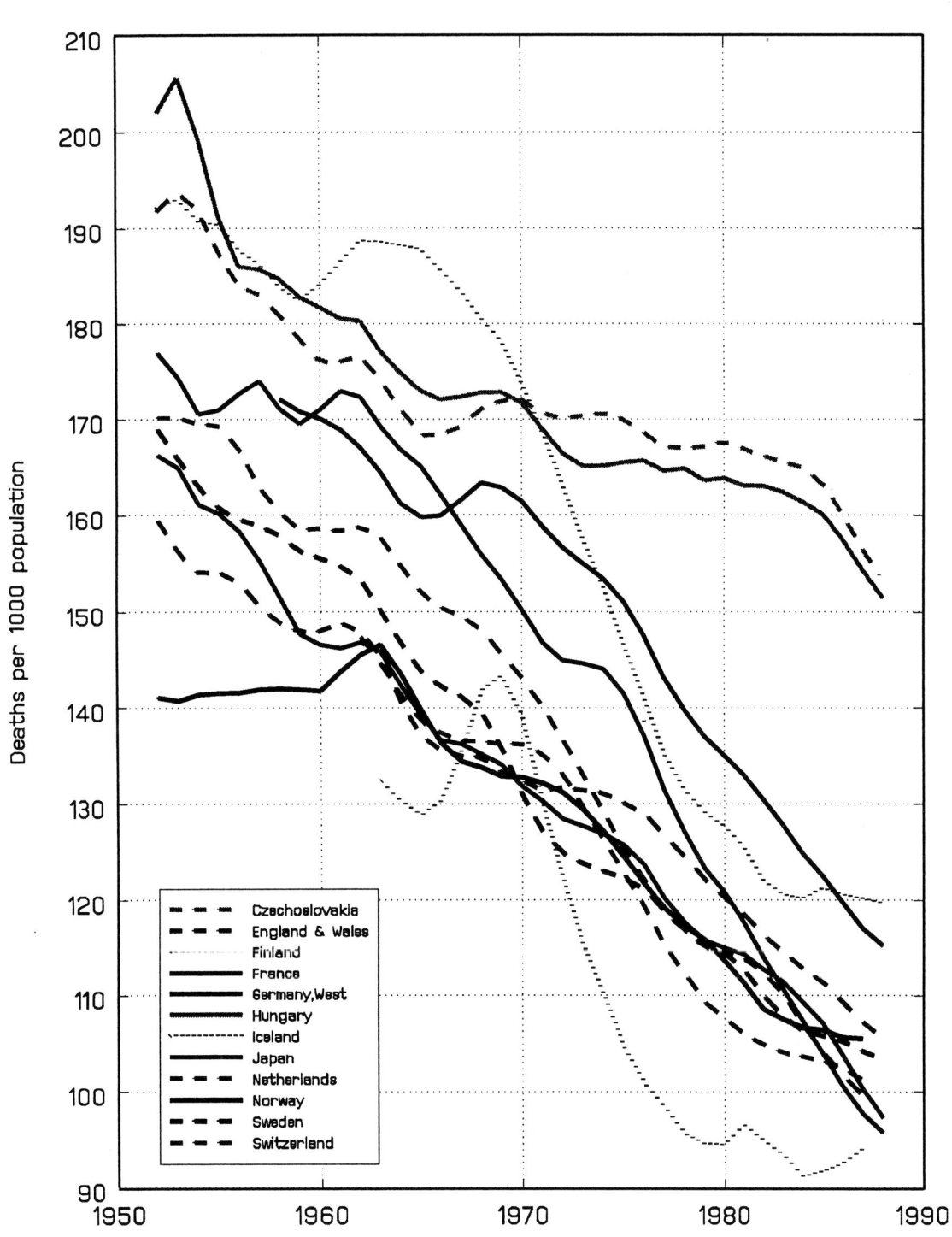

A glance at these graphs leaves no doubt about the generalized decline of mortality in the post-war period but also makes clear the existence of widely varying speeds, some sluggish, some precipitous, as well as the occurrence of periods of short-term increase here and there.

In the tumultuous development the curves of different countries often cross each other, sometimes only to recross soon after, sometimes signifying a more permanent change in ranking. It may further be appreciated that in a general way the curves have been falling more steeply in the second half of the period, roughly after 1970. This testifies to a tendency of the decline to accelerate, and this acceleration is percentage-wise even sharper than shown in the arithmetic scale of the figure. A comparison of the two figures shows further that the decline of mortality has been more pronounced among women than men. In fact, a more thorough examination of the figures and the underlying data in the Annex will show that there has been no exception to the faster mortality decline for women and that even in the countries of the former East bloc where male mortality long remained stationary, the female rates showed significant improvement. Among the 26 countries listed in Table 6 and showing death rates for two separate dates, the unweighted mean of mortality decline was 14.4 percent for males and 25.7 percent for females.

It may be asked whether it is possible to reduce the large variety of national time series into a smaller number of scenarios, each of which has prevailed in several countries. We shall try to do this by considering both the level and the speed of decline in each country.

Although in the global context all countries of the database are low-mortality countries, there are between them differences large enough to discern the existence of high-, medium- and low-mortality groups among them. Some countries, however, do not conform to any of these groups while some others have during the observation period moved from one group to another.

Finally, a few countries defy precise classification because of uncertainty about the data. The six-way classification below is therefore not very clear-cut but may be of some help in the examination of this particular mortality history. In reading the comments the reader may refer to Figure 2(a,b), to country-wise data in Table 6 and aggregate rates in Table 7. Further details are given in Annex Tables 2, 3 and 4.

Table 6.   AGE-STANDARDIZED DEATH RATES AT AGES 80-99 IN 1955-59 AND 1985-89.
            TOTAL AND ANNUAL DECLINE

Country	Males				Females			
	Deaths per 1000		Decline %		Deaths per 1000		Decline %	
	1955-1959	1985-1989	Total	p.a.	1955-1959	1985-1989	Total	p.a.
Australia	177.3	143.2	19.2	1.1	133.2	98.8	25.8	1.5
Austria	201.9	162.3	19.6	0.7	171.7	128.5	25.2	1.0
Belgium	193.8	163.0	15.5	0.6	165.8	115.8	30.2	1.2
Czechoslovakia	207.4	197.7	4.7	0.2	181.8	157.0	13.6	0.5
Denmark	172.4	149.0	13.6	0.5	157.2	105.8	32.7	1.3
England & Wales	200.3	159.3	20.5	0.8	151.6	108.1	28.7	1.1
Estonia	189.1	179.5	5.1	0.2	157.9	140.2	11.2	0.4
Finland	209.0	161.9	22.5	0.8	186.4	121.0	35.1	1.4
France	197.0	145.9	25.9	1.0	154.6	100.9	34.7	1.4
Germany, East	199.0	199.7	- 0.4	- 0.0	178.0	157.9	11.3	0.4
Germany, West	194.7	161.8	16.9	0.6	171.0	117.6	31.2	1.2
Hungary	200.5	195.8	2.3	0.1	184.0	154.7	15.9	0.6
Iceland	154.8	125.4	19.0	0.9	133.8	94.8	29.1	1.4
Ireland	190.8	174.5	8.5	0.3	161.8	127.1	21.4	0.8
Italy	176.7	152.2	13.9	0.5	153.8	113.1	26.5	1.0
Japan	209.6	137.6	34.4	1.4	170.3	98.0	42.5	1.8
Latvia	172.3	174.7	- 1.4	- 0.0	139.9	139.1	0.6	0.0
Luxemburg	209.1	175.7	16.0	0.6	174.9	121.1	30.8	1.2
Netherlands	163.8	150.7	8.0	0.3	145.9	101.9	30.2	1.4
New Zealand	168.4	155.8	7.5	0.3	137.4	111.4	18.9	0.7
Norway	153.4	147.8	3.7	0.1	141.6	105.9	25.2	1.0
Poland	178.7	186.0	- 4.1	- 0.3	145.2	147.7	- 1.7	- 0.1
Portugal	207.5	170.5	17.8	0.7	164.2	131.7	19.8	0.7
Scotland	210.1	174.6	16.9	0.6	171.0	119.4	30.2	1.2
Singapore	...	132.0	...	...	...	103.7	...	...
Spain	187.4	140.7	25.1	1.0	153.1	113.7	25.7	1.0
Sweden	174.9	149.5	14.5	0.5	157.4	104.2	33.4	1.4
Switzerland	190.6	142.3	25.3	1.0	163.6	99.8	39.0	1.6
Aggregates:								
- High mortality 3 countries	201.6	198.3	1.6	0.1	180.3	157.0	12.9	0.5
- Medium mort. 5 countries	196.5	160.8	18.2	0.7	162.1	114.2	29.5	1.2
- Low mortality 4 countries	169.3	150.4	11.2	0.4	153.7	104.4	32.1	1.3
- Rapid decline 2 countries	196.5	145.6	25.9	1.0	155.4	94.8	39.0	1.6
- W.Europe 11 countries	192.7	155.2	19.5	0.7	159.0	109.1	31.4	1.2

The following periods were substituted: Australia 1965-69 for 1955-59; Iceland 1961-64 for 1955-59; Netherlands 1960-64 for 1955-59; Poland 1971-74 for 1955-59; Spain 1985-86 for 1985-89.

(i) Iceland

Iceland has had and continues to have the lowest reliably recorded mortality at old age in the world. The advance over other countries is particularly notable among men. The population being small, annual rates are volatile but substantial mortality decline is nevertheless obvious and has amounted to 25 percent in as many years.

Table 7. AGE-STANDARDIZED DEATH RATES 80-99 YEARS IN GROUPS OF COUNTRIES

Sex and period	Low mortality group	Rapid decline group	Medium mortality group	High mortality group	Western Europe
Males					
1950-54	175.18	206.70	...	...	...
1955-59	169.31	196.48	196.46	201.57	192.73
1960-64	169.81	188.21	193.19	203.36	188.73
1965-69	163.97	179.33	189.47	204.94	183.28
1970-74	158.56	170.16	186.93	203.00	178.51
1975-79	155.89	165.99	182.43	204.35	174.34
1980-84	151.87	157.76	171.52	206.68	165.08
1985-89	150.35	145.63	160.85	198.33	155.20
Females					
1950-54	163.95	165.65	...	...	...
1955-59	153.73	155.39	162.07	180.28	158.96
1960-64	150.25	146.65	157.71	178.62	153.63
1965-69	139.99	137.74	151.06	175.33	145.87
1970-74	129.01	129.26	145.80	172.44	138.95
1975-79	117.90	120.49	136.85	168.45	129.77
1980-84	108.65	112.57	124.46	165.27	119.05
1985-89	104.36	100.81	114.17	156.99	109.13

Low-mortality group: Denmark, Netherlands, Norway, Sweden.
Rapid-decline group: France, Switzerland.
Medium-mortality group: Austria, Belgium, England & Wales, Finland, Germany (West).
High-mortality group: Czechoslovakia, Germany (East), Hungary.
Western Europe: Aggregate of the three first-mentioned groups.

The good quality of the data is highlighted by a list of all centenarians since 1950, prepared by the national statistical office Hagstofa Islands, giving for each one the name, sex, place of residence, date of birth, date of death (if deceased) and the age reached (years, months, days).

(ii) Japan

Japan has the distinction of having experienced in the post-war era the sharpest decline in old age mortality among all the countries of the database: 39.8 percent in 30 years. Old age mortality was quite high in Japan until about 1960 when it began to fall extremely fast. This has continued ever since so that at the latest date on record Japan is in the forefront of the low-mortality countries though still some distance behind Iceland.

(iii) Low-mortality group

This group includes four countries with traditionally low mortality. *Norway* and the *Netherlands* recorded already before 1950 particularly low death rates which were almost as low for men as for women. In the period that followed, the male rates have made only slight progress (3.7 and 8.0 percent respectively) and have been overtaken by several other countries. The development of the female rates has been more favourable with declines of 25.2 and 30.2 but even these have lost some ground in relation to a few other countries.

Sweden and *Denmark*, the latter not shown in the figures, belong naturally and even geographically to the same group. Beginning with slightly higher, though internationally quite low rates, they have recorded more sustained decline amounting to about 14 percent for men and 33 percent for women. The result has been that the mortality in the four countries has converged to a solid low level.

(iv) Rapid decline group

Switzerland and *France* are characterized by a very regular, rapid and sustained decline of mortality over the entire post-war period which has amounted to 34.4 and 31.8 percent respectively, results exceeded only by Japan. The improvement has been remarkable also for men: more than 25 percent. Although starting at moderately high level in the 1950s, their death rates are now among the lowest on record. For women they are already consistently below the 100 mark, only slightly above those of Iceland and Japan.

(v) Medium-mortality group

This group, larger and less uniform than the others, is headed by *England and Wales* where the mortality of women has been approximately on the Scandinavian level while that of men, considerably higher, has kept the combined rate above that of the low-mortality group. The decline, though regular and substantial (26.0 percent), has been slower than e.g. in France causing the English rates to fall gradually behind.

The position of England and Wales is closely matched by *Italy* which, however, has a lower death rate for men but a higher one for women. Italy is not shown in the figures because its data for the first post-war decades were apparently affected by age overstatement and the actual decline may have been faster than the calculated 22.3 percent.

Next in this group are *Belgium* (not shown in figures), *West Germany* and *Finland*, their respective rates of decline having been 25.3, 26.4 and 30.9 percent. Most of this decline took place in Finland after 1970 and in West Germany after 1975, being therefore remarkably rapid for a short period and showing now signs of slowing down.

Slightly higher death rates are recorded for *Scotland*, *Austria* and *Luxemburg* which are not shown graphically. Scotland, like England, is characterized by an unusually high excess mortality of men. The three countries have posted good average declines of close to 25 percent or roughly one percent per year. Among the men the progress gained momentum only in the late 1970s but has been rapid since then.

In the same group, though with again somewhat higher rates, we have included *Portugal* and *Ireland*. In these countries the apparent progress has been slower (19 and 17 percent respectively) but this may be an artifact caused by improving data quality.

(vi) High mortality group

This group is composed by six countries of the former East bloc. The data for *Czechoslovakia*, *East Germany* and *Hungary* are of proven good quality and can be used for describing the entire group. The death rates calculated for these countries - closely similar for all three - are the highest in the entire study. The apparent rates for *Estonia*, *Latvia* and *Poland* are lower but unreliable due to considerable age overstatement which in the case of Estonia and probably also of Latvia has been caused by Soviet immigrants.

The group is represented in Figures 2a and 2b by only Czechoslovakia and Hungary because the curves for East Germany would be almost indistinguishable from them. The male curves show stagnation and even increase until a very recent turn for the better. For women, more sustained but sluggish improvement can be noted. The overall declines are the lowest in the database except for the questionable data for Latvia and Poland which would indicate a slight increase.

(vii) Other countries

The scenarios for a few other countries are more difficult to assess and classify. *Australia* seems to belong at present to the low-mortality group even though the exact level of mortality there may not be accurately represented by the calculated death rates. The past developments in Australia are also somewhat in doubt, not least because we have the requisite data only from 1965. What can be considered certain is that a declining trend has been operating there too. *New Zealand* non-Maoris display medium-level death rates and belong no doubt to the medium-mortality group of populations even if the calculated rates would not be very precise. More uncertain is the past course of mortality which according to the data has been one of only slow decline. The data for the *Singapore* Chinese indicate low mortality but the series available is still too short for a definitive assessment. The use of the Chinese calendar is hoped to assure reliable information on age.

The data for *Spain* suggest quite low mortality already some time ago but are obviously biased by considerable age overstatement. This is to an even greater extent the case of *Canada*, *Chile* and the *New Zealand* Maoris.

During the last 30 years the ranking of the countries regarding mortality level has undergone an extensive transformation as is evident from Table 8 and Figure 3.

In this comparison we have included only the 19 countries with good quality data plus Ireland and Portugal in which the death rates calculated for at least the 1985-89 period can be considered fairly precise.

The change has been so deep-going that most of the countries have moved down to levels apparently never reached before. The lowest rate of the 1950s would now be one of the highest in Western Europe. At the same time the ranking of the countries has changed thoroughly. Only the leading position of Iceland has not been seriously challenged but Norway and the Netherlands have ceded their places to rapidly advancing Japan, Switzerland and France.

Finland, Scotland and Luxemburg have moved from their former lagging positions close to the middle while Portugal, Ireland and Austria have been pressed relatively more back in spite of large reductions in mortality.

Table 8.   RANKING OF COUNTRIES ACCORDING TO MORTALITY AT AGES 80-99 IN 1955-59 AND 1985-89. BOTH SEXES.

Age-standardized death rate per 1000 population			
1955-59		1985-89	
Iceland	140.8	Iceland	105.0
Norway	145.5	Japan	111.2
Netherlands	151.9	Switzerland	114.0
Italy	161.4	France	115.9
Denmark	162.3	Netherlands	118.2
Sweden	163.2	Sweden	119.3
England & Wales	167.8	Norway	119.9
France	168.7	Denmark	120.2
Ireland	171.5	England & Wales	125.2
Switzerland	172.6	Italy	126.1
Belgium	175.1	Belgium	131.5
Portugal	178.6	Germany, West	132.3
Germany, West	179.3	Finland	134.6
Austria	181.8	Scotland	137.8
Japan	183.4	Luxemburg	139.3
Scotland	184.0	Austria	139.8
Germany, East	185.0	Ireland	142.5
Hungary	185.9	Portugal	144.6
Luxemburg	186.3	Hungary	168.4
Czechoslovakia	190.3	Czechoslovakia	170.6
Finland	193.9	Germany, East	171.8

The following periods were substituted: Iceland 1961-64 for 1955-59; Netherlands 1960-64 for 1955-59.

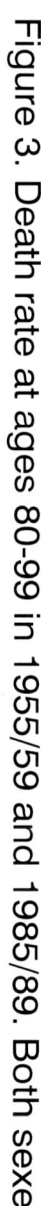

Figure 3. Death rate at ages 80-99 in 1955/59 and 1985/89. Both sexes.

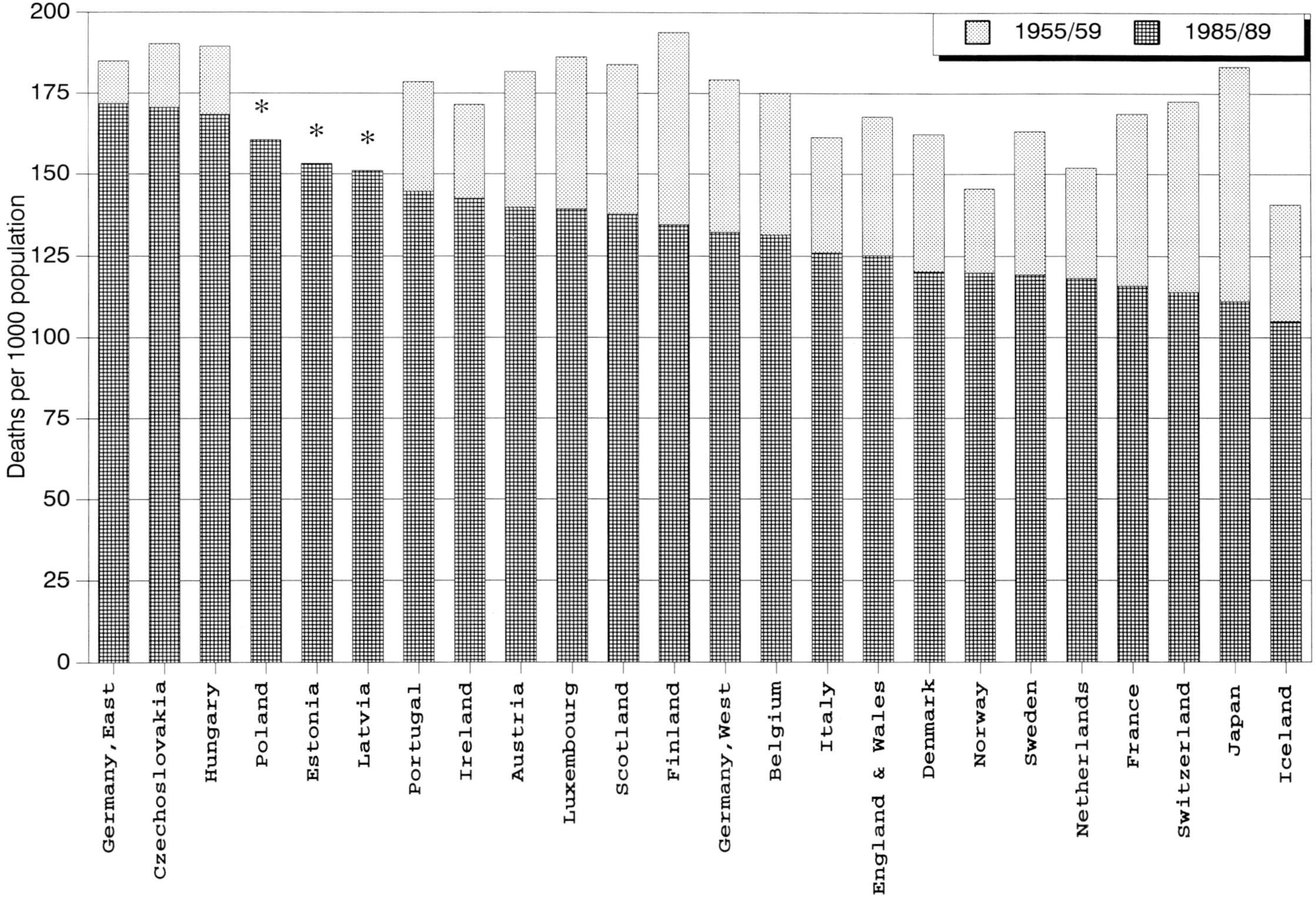

* - Rates in 1955/59 not reliably known for Poland, Estonia and Latvia

The shake-out has left East Germany, Czechoslovakia and Hungary at the end although even there, reductions in death rates, mainly of women, have taken place. The rates calculated for Poland (160.5), Estonia (153.3) and Latvia (151.0) would place them in the next lowest ranks but they are believed to be affected by age errors and are not included in the table.

The development has not led to greater similarity but, on the contrary, to wider differentiation. While the unweighted mean for the 21 countries fell from 172.8 to 132.7, the standard deviation rose from 14.3 to 19.2 and the coefficient of variation from 8.3 to 14.5. This was mainly caused by the East-West divergence but even if the former East bloc countries are excluded, the coefficient of variation has grown from 8.4 to 9.3.

The development of mortality by sex is given for each country in Table 9 and in Figure 4. In all countries without exception the development has been more favourable to females than males, thus increasing the already existing gender gap of mortality. In Portugal and Spain this additional element has been very small while in the other extreme the Netherlands and Norway have seen widely different development for the two sexes and in Eastern Europe the progress has been essentially limited to women only.

The data for aggregates summarize this development: (i) hardly any improvement for men in the high-mortality group; (ii) sharply differential progress in favour of women in the traditional low-mortality countries; (iii) rapid decline has been possible only when also men have fully taken part in it: the case of Switzerland and France is strengthened by evidence from Japan and Finland.

The decline of mortality has up to now been mainly discussed in relative terms which is perhaps the more common viewpoint of observers in general. The demographic impact, however, can be better judged by the changes in relation to population. In these terms, per 1000 population of both sexes, aged 80-99, the following declines were recorded between 1955-59 and 1985-89 (as given in Table 9):

Table 9. DECLINE OF MORTALITY AT AGES 80-99 FROM 1955-59 TO 1985-89.

Country	Percent			Per 1000 population		
	Total	Male	Female	Total	Male	Female
Australia	23.6	19.2	25.8	34.3	34.1	34.4
Austria	23.1	19.6	25.2	42.0	39.6	43.2
Belgium	24.9	15.9	30.2	43.6	30.8	50.0
Czechoslovakia	10.4	4.7	13.6	19.7	9.7	24.8
Denmark	25.9	13.6	32.7	42.1	23.4	51.4
England & Wales	25.4	20.5	28.7	42.6	41.0	43.5
Estonia	9.2	5.1	11.2	15.0	9.6	17.7
Finland	30.6	22.5	35.1	59.3	47.1	65.4
France	31.3	25.9	34.7	52.8	51.1	53.7
Germany, East	7.1	- 0.4	11.3	13.2	- 0.7	20.1
Germany, West	26.2	16.9	31.5	47.0	32.9	54.0
Hungary	11.1	2.3	15.9	21.1	4.7	29.3
Iceland	25.5	19.0	29.1	35.8	29.4	39.0
Ireland	16.9	8.5	21.4	29.0	16.3	34.7
Italy	21.9	13.9	26.5	35.3	24.5	40.7
Japan	39.4	34.4	42.5	72.2	72.0	72.3
Latvia	- 0.1	- 1.4	0.6	- 0.3	- 2.4	0.8
Luxemburg	25.2	16.0	30.8	47.0	33.4	53.8
Netherlands	22.2	8.0	30.2	33.7	13.1	44.0
New Zealand	15.1	7.5	18.9	21.5	12.6	26.0
Norway	17.6	3.7	25.2	25.6	5.6	35.7
Poland	- 2.5	- 4.1	- 1.7	- 4.1	- 7.3	- 2.5
Portugal	19.0	17.8	19.8	34.0	37.0	32.5
Scotland	25.1	16.9	30.2	46.2	35.5	51.6
Singapore	...	...	...	...	...	...
Spain	25.5	25.1	25.7	41.8	46.7	39.4
Sweden	26.9	14.5	33.8	43.9	25.4	53.2
Switzerland	34.0	25.3	39.0	58.6	48.3	63.8
Aggregates:						
- High mortality 3 countries	9.1	1.6	12.9	16.6	3.3	23.3
- Medium mortal. 5 countries	25.7	18.2	29.5	43.8	35.7	47.9
- Low mortality 4 countries	25.1	11.2	32.1	39.2	18.9	49.3
- Rapid decline 2 countries	34.6	25.9	39.0	57.4	50.9	60.6
- Western Europe 11 countries	27.4	19.5	31.4	45.8	37.5	49.9

Certain time periods have been substituted in some countries as in Table 6.

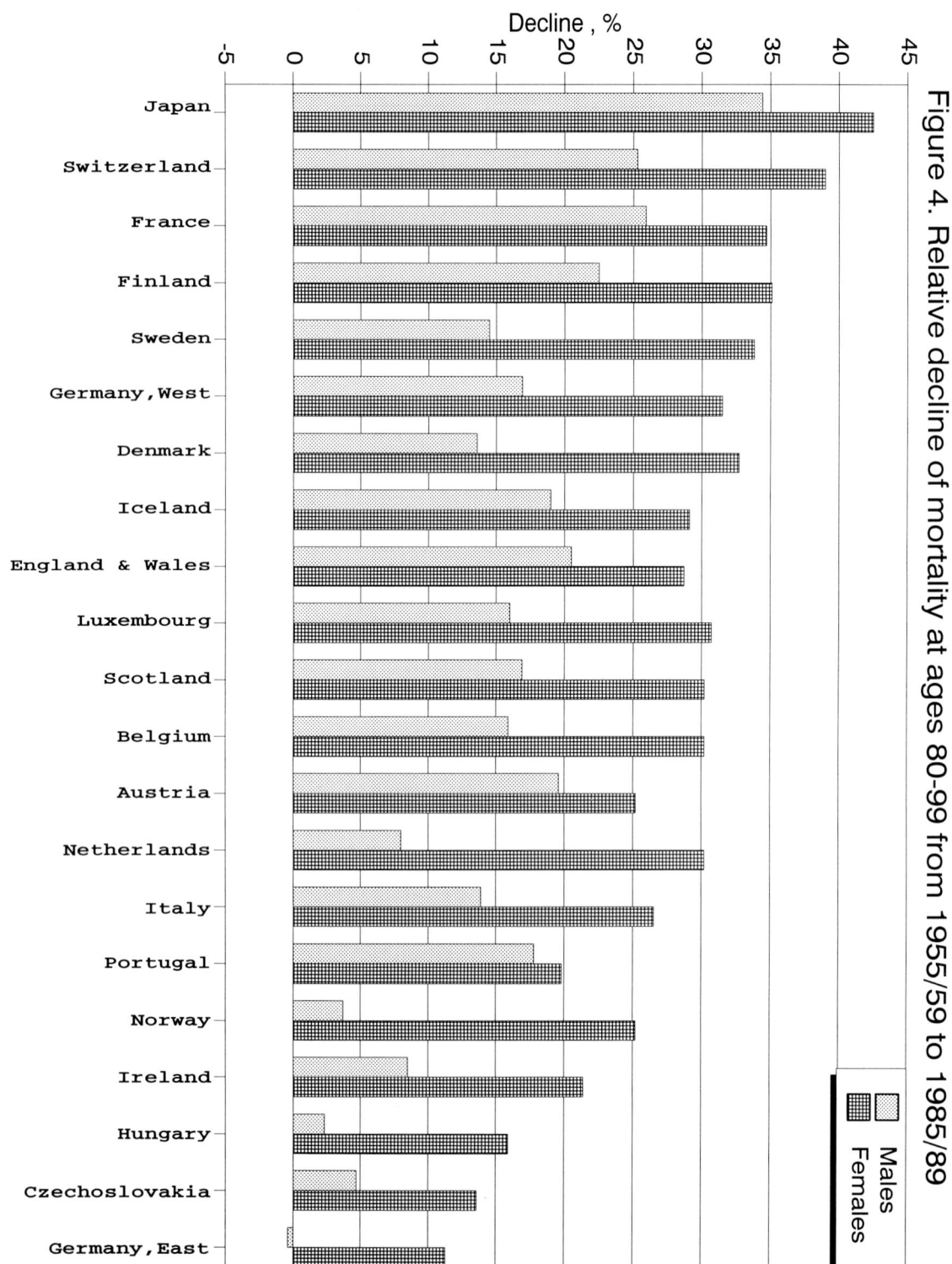

Figure 4. Relative decline of mortality at ages 80-99 from 1955/59 to 1985/89

Japan	72.2	Italy	35.3
Finland	59.3	Australia	34.3
Switzerland	58.6	Portugal	34.0
France	52.8	Netherlands	33.7
Germany, West	47.0	Ireland	29.0
Luxemburg	47.0	Norway	25.6
Scotland	46.2	New Zealand	21.5
Sweden	43.9	Hungary	21.1
Belgium	43.6	Czechoslovakia	19.7
England & Wales	42.6	Estonia	15.0
Denmark	42.1	Germany, East	13.2
Austria	42.0	Latvia	- 0.3
Spain	41.8	Poland	- 4.1
Iceland	35.8		

The decline that has taken place in Japan is also in this comparison outstanding. Finland, Switzerland and France have undergone the greatest reductions in Europe while also the gains made in West Germany, Luxemburg and Scotland are impressive. Many other changes in ranking when compared with percentage decline have also taken place. The six countries of the former East bloc remain nevertheless at the end of the list.

9. *Onset of sustained mortality decline*

From what has been said above it is clear that though a decline in old age mortality has taken place internationally on a very broad front, it did not begin simultaneously everywhere. We shall now try to pinpoint for each country and sex the time of onset of sustained decline. For this purpose we have calculated the 5-year means of the age-adjusted death rate at ages 80-99 in the manner of moving averages but assigning each mean to the last of the 5 years involved. These values are given in Annex Table 6.

We may consider the year of onset of the decline to be the earliest year in which the 5-year mean fell to a level which it never exceeded again and after which the decline was never significantly broken by an increase or a period of see-saw rates.

This rule allows some fluctuation in annual death rates but no significant break in the declining trend. Using this criterion, the years of onset of sustained mortality decline are those given in Table 10.

Among the 25 countries in which it could be determined, the onset varied a great deal and took place generally much earlier for females than males, the average time difference being eight years. Exceptions in which the male rate began to decline first are few and not significant.

France is unique in that mortality decline has been continuous there for the entire period starting therefore already in 1955 or earlier for both sexes. Two of its neighbours, Switzerland and Belgium, also had early starts.

Table 10.   ONSET OF SUSTAINED DECLINE IN OLD-AGE MORTALITY

Country	Female	Male
France	1955[1]	1955[1]
Switzerland	1956	1967
Belgium	1956	1978
Sweden	1956	1978
Denmark	1962	1984
England & Wales	1964	1977
Scotland	1964	1977
Netherlands	1965	1977
Japan	1966	1966
Finland	1967	1970
Norway	1968	1974
Portugal	1970	1970
Australia	1970	1975
Italy	1970	1978
Luxemburg	1970	1979
Germany, West	1971	1973
Austria	1972	1976
Iceland	1972	1984
Hungary	1972	1985
Germany, East	1973	1984
Spain	1974	1972
New Zealand	1974	1973
Czechoslovakia	1975	1985
Ireland	1979	1978
Estonia	1981	1989
Mean	1968	1976

[1] Or earlier.
No sustained decline could be determined for Latvia, Poland or Singapore.

In late 1960s the decline began to reach wider areas and by 1970s it had become almost universal in low-mortality countries.

The onset of the remarkably rapid decline in Japan was not very early and can be timed to 1966 for both sexes. In countries of traditionally low mortality (Scandinavia and the Netherlands), female death rates entered a sustained decline already in the 1950s or 1960s while the male rates showed resistance till much later, and in Denmark turned decisively down only in the 1980s.

It can be observed that the decline began simultaneously in England and Wales and in Scotland, and that Austria followed West Germany with only a small time lag. In the former East bloc, female rates began to decline in the 1970s but male rates only around 1985, if at all. In Latvia and Poland, mortality has not yet entered a definitely declining stage and they are therefore excluded from the table, as is Singapore for which the observed period is still too short.

Table 11 gives an overview of the *speed* of the mortality decline in each country during the period in which it has proceeded in a sustained fashion. The speed is indicated in the table in terms of annual percent decline, measured for each year by the mean rate for the last five years compared with the mean of the five years preceding them. It therefore gives the mean decline during the last ten years.

We can observe several countries with relatively even rates of decline for females, in some quite rapid, as in France and Sweden, in others more moderate, as in England and Wales, Scotland, Italy and Norway, or frankly sluggish as in the former East bloc. In several other countries the trend has clearly accelerated over time and among these are Switzerland, Japan, Belgium, West Germany and Austria while in some others, such as Denmark, the Netherlands and Finland, rapid acceleration has been followed by a slowdown. The most precipitous decline, exceeding 4 percent per year was experienced by Icelandic women in the 1970s.

The rates of decline have been notably slower for males and no 10-year period with a sustained drop of 3 percent per year has been observed. However, also here we can frequently note an acceleration of the decline which in some cases has later slowed down but in others is continuing apace.

This examination confirms the existence of a generalized mortality decline of recent origin but with considerable geographical variation as to its onset, speed, acceleration and occasional slowdown.

Table 11. ANNUAL DECLINE OF MORTALITY AT AGES 80-99. CALCULATED FROM THE MEAN FOR THE LAST 5 YEARS RELATIVE TO THE MEAN FOR THE PRECEDING 5 YEARS.

FEMALES

Country	1955-1959	1960-1964	1965-1969	1970-1974	1975-1979	1980-1984	1985-1989	1990
France	00001	11111	10011	11101	01111	11111	11112	2
Switzerland	0000	01100	00011	01111	22222	22111	11122	2
Belgium	0000	01100	00000	00000	01111	12221	11112	2
Sweden	0001	00000	11111	11122	21110	01111	11111	1
Denmark		000	00011	12332	21111	11100	00010	1
England & Wales		0	00111	11000	00000	01111	11111	1
Scotland		0	11221	11001	10000	01111	10110	1
Netherlands			00001	11000	11222	22221	11100	
Japan			0011	11111	11112	22332	22223	2
Finland			000	11112	22333	33221	11100	0
Norway			01	11100	00111	11111	11110	0
Portugal				00000	00000	11111	11000	0
Australia				00000	11112	22222	11110	1
Italy				00012	11000	01111	11122	
Luxemburg				00011	11101	12211	11122	
Germany, West				0000	01111	22222	11121	1
Austria				000	00100	00111	11111	2
Iceland				001	34444	32210	0100+	
Hungary				000	00000	00000	00001	1
Germany, East				00	00100	00000	00000	1
Spain				0	00011	22222	11	
New Zealand				0	00111	12110	0000+	0
Czechoslovakia					00000	0000+	00001	1
Ireland					0	01111	11110	
Estonia						0000	000+0	0

0 = less than 1 percent
1 = 1 - 2 percent
2 = 2 - 3 percent
3 = 3 - 4 percent
4 = 4 percent or more
+ = increase

e.g. the third figure for Denmark in 1970-74 is 3. It corresponds to year 1972 and indicates that the death rate in 1968-72 shows a mean annual decline of 3-4 percent in relation to 1963-67.

Table 11 (cont.).   ANNUAL DECLINE OF MORTALITY AT AGES 80-99.

MALES

Country	1955-1959	1960-1964	1965-1969	1970-1974	1975-1979	1980-1984	1985-1989	1990
France	00001	11100	00101	10001	00000	01111	00011	2
Japan			0011	11111	11112	22221	11111	1
Switzerland			000	01011	11111	11000	01111	1
Finland				00001	11212	11211	11000	0
Portugal				00000	00000	01111	10000	0
Spain				000	00011	22222	11	
Germany, West				00	00000	11111	11111	1
New Zealand				00	00000	00100	10000	
Norway				0	00000	00000	00000	0
Australia					00001	12221	10110	1
Austria					0000	00011	11122	2
England & Wales					000	01001	10111	1
Netherlands					000	01000	0++++	0
Scotland					000	00000	00110	0
Belgium					00	11100	00011	1
Sweden					00	00000	00000	0
Italy					00	00001	11111	
Ireland					0+	+0000	00000	
Luxemburg					0	00111	10000	
Denmark						0	00000	0
Iceland						0	+0010	
Germany, East						0	+0000	0
Czechoslovakia							00011	1
Hungary							00000	1
Estonia							0	0

0 = less than 1 percent
1 = 1 - 2 percent
2 = 2 - 3 percent
3 = 3 - 4 percent
4 = 4 percent or more
+ = increase

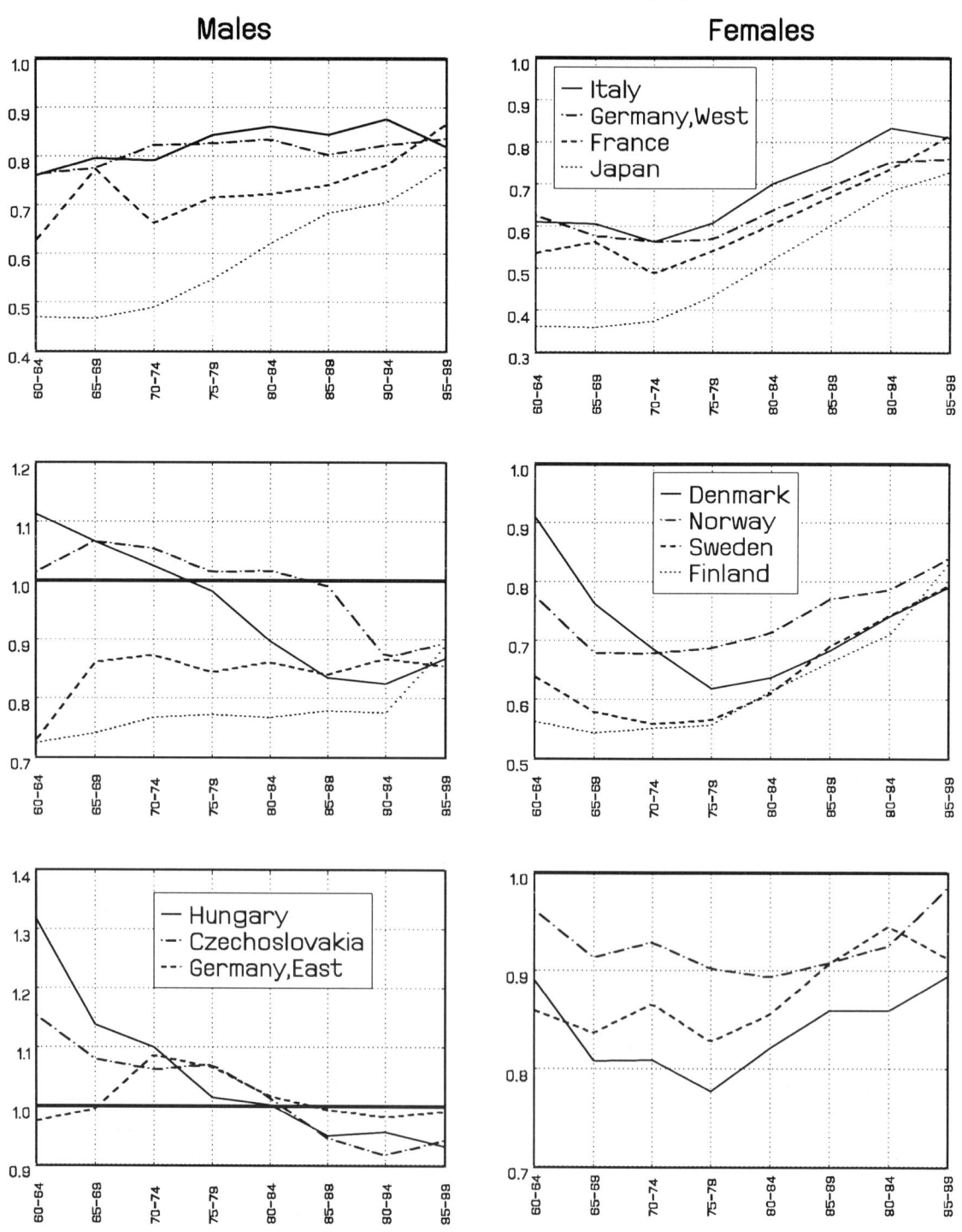

Figure 5. Relative change of mortality by age and sex from 1955-59 to 1985-89.

Data below age 80 are based on U.N. Demographic Yearbook.

10. Age pattern of mortality decline

10.1. The elderly in 12 selected countries

In order to provide a better perspective on the age pattern of recent mortality changes among the oldest-old, we give in the following first an overview of the changes observed among the elderly in general from age 60 up. The data for the age bracket 60-79 have been drawn from various editions of the United Nations Demographic Yearbook and refer approximately to the periods 1955-59 and 1985-89 (the death rates in certain years in some countries were not published). From them, percentage decline was calculated for quinquennial age groups in the interval 60-84 years in twelve selected countries and the series was extended to older quinquennial age groups using data from our database and verification showed that the two sources agreed well in the pivotal age group 80-84. The results are given in Annex Table 6 and Figure 5. Because of small numbers the ratios for centenarians are given in the table only for the largest countries and, being rather erratic, are not reproduced in the figure.

The results for males reveal striking differences between countries. The first frame shows considerable but differential progress in four large countries. The very deep decline in both Japan and France has been strongly age-selective and the younger elderly have made much greater gains than the oldest. The more moderate gains in West Germany and Italy do not adhere to this pattern beyond age 80: among the very oldest they are nearly as large as among sexagenarians.

In the Netherlands (not shown in the figure) the age pattern has a shape similar to that in West Germany and Italy but the curve moves on a higher level and the death rates of the 70-79-year-old have actually risen.

The Nordic countries show even greater divergence. In Finland a very substantial progress has followed the age pattern of France while the gains in Sweden have been almost non-selective. In Denmark and Norway the mortality of the younger elderly has increased and only the oldest-old show declining rates.

In the Central European countries of the former East bloc the development has been quite alarming. The mortality of the younger elderly men has increased sharply and only the 85-and-over have seen any improvement at all.

It is perhaps expected that mortality can be more easily reduced among relatively younger people than the very oldest. This expectation is met in the data for men in Japan, France and Finland. The data for West Germany, Italy and Sweden are roughly neutral in this respect showing no clear dependency on age.

In the Netherlands gains are recorded among the youngest elderly and again among the oldest. Finally, Norway, Denmark and the former East bloc countries show a contrasting picture where the younger elderly have not benefited at all and the gains have been largest among the oldest.

The data on women present an entirely different, more regular and uniform picture. Although the size of the gains does vary considerably between countries, they are in all cases gradually reduced as age increases. The largest gains, though, have not taken place at the youngest ages but in the upper sixties or the seventies. After this, the gains have narrowed down with age in all twelve countries.

10.2 The oldest-old in 28 countries

In the narrower age band of the oldest-old the Odense database allows relatively accurate description of the changes in a number of countries as brought together in Table 12. The figures for some of them should, however, be regarded with caution. Besides the weaknesses in the basic data in a few countries as pointed out before, the rates for Iceland and Luxemburg are in this table affected by the small numbers involved. Steadier time series by age group are given in Annex Table 7 for aggregates of countries in quinquennial periods.

The existence, among men, of sharp contrasts in the age pattern of mortality decline, noted above between 12 countries, is confirmed on a broader front. The expected diminishing gains with advancing age can be seen, in addition to Japan, France and Finland, unequivocally also in Australia, Austria, Portugal and Switzerland and somewhat less clearly in Ireland and Scotland. It deserves to be noted that all the countries where the overall gains have been the largest - Japan, France, Switzerland and Finland - share this same age pattern of change.

Roughly equal mortality decline at all ages can be seen in Belgium, England and Wales, Germany (West), Italy, New Zealand and Sweden, and the same is suggested by the data for Spain.

In sharp contrast to all the above, the men in the Netherlands and Norway have registered only small, if any, gains around age 80 (at ages 70-79 the mortality increased) and substantial benefits have accrued only to the very oldest. It will be recalled that in these two countries the mortality of old men has been traditionally low. The shape of the curve is basically similar in Denmark. The modest gains made in the former East bloc also tend to concentrate in oldest ages.

Looking at the figures for the aggregates at the bottom of Table 12 we note that the gains increase with age in the low-mortality group, decline with age in the rapid decline group, the two tendencies are cancelled out in the medium-mortality group

Table 12.   DECLINE OF MORTALITY BY AGE AND SEX FROM 1955-59 TO 1985-89, PERCENT.

Country	Males				Females			
	80-84	85-89	90-94	95-99	80-84	85-89	90-94	95-99
Australia	20.0	20.9	13.5	11.3	28.2	27.0	18.3	11.0
Austria	20.2	19.8	17.7	16.3	29.3	23.6	16.7	16.2
Belgium	14.5	16.5	19.6	16.3	33.3	29.1	23.8	22.7
Czechoslovakia	1.1	8.5	10.6	- 6.6	14.2	13.7	13.2	5.6
Denmark	10.3	16.6	17.6	13.3	36.3	31.7	25.8	20.9
England & Wales	19.0	22.1	22.0	21.1	30.8	28.6	22.9	22.0
Estonia	5.8	6.0	- 0.9	6.1	11.7	11.1	11.4	2.1
Finland	23.3	22.2	22.5	11.2	38.7	33.8	29.1	17.0
France	27.8	25.9	21.8	13.5	39.6	33.0	26.4	18.4
Germany, East	- 1.7	0.6	1.8	0.9	14.5	9.3	5.5	8.7
Germany, West	16.5	19.7	17.7	16.4	36.3	30.5	24.7	23.9
Hungary	- 0.2	5.0	4.4	6.8	17.9	14.1	14.1	10.6
Iceland	17.6	24.8	7.7	22.0	34.4	23.4	27.5	13.4
Ireland	9.8	12.3	- 2.5	- 9.4	24.6	22.1	10.5	8.3
Italy	12.7	15.4	12.4	19.0	31.2	24.3	17.3	18.8
Japan	38.0	31.5	29.5	22.1	48.2	39.9	31.7	27.3
Latvia	- 5.3	1.0	6.2	- 0.8	3.6	- 0.6	- 5.4	- 12.6
Luxemburg	13.3	14.1	31.5	4.6	30.5	36.1	18.2	23.1
Netherlands	4.9	9.1	13.3	20.5	34.3	28.7	22.0	21.6
New Zealand	7.6	9.4	1.2	11.5	21.7	19.7	7.6	16.8
Norway	- 1.7	6.0	13.1	10.6	28.7	23.0	21.4	16.1
Poland	- 3.2	- 6.2	- 2.7	2.9	2.7	- 6.0	- 5.7	- 6.7
Portugal	18.9	17.7	15.3	12.2	22.1	17.8	16.0	20.8
Scotland	16.7	17.9	15.4	15.4	32.3	29.5	24.9	28.9
Singapore	...	...	...	...	...	...	...	...
Spain	26.4	25.3	19.0	25.9	32.3	23.0	9.9	12.8
Sweden	13.9	16.0	13.3	14.6	39.1	31.0	25.7	20.7
Switzerland	26.9	28.0	15.2	13.3	44.4	37.9	27.4	20.6
Aggregates:								
- High mortality 3 countries	- 0.5	3.7	4.8	0.1	15.1	11.5	9.5	8.3
- Medium mortal. 5 countries	17.8	20.5	19.8	18.3	33.5	29.3	23.5	22.5
- Low mortality 4 countries	8.1	13.5	15.1	16.1	36.3	30.2	25.3	21.0
- Rapid decline 2 countries	27.8	26.0	21.2	13.5	40.0	33.5	26.4	18.6
- Western Europe 11 countries	19.5	21.3	19.6	16.8	35.6	30.5	24.5	21.2

Time periods have been substituted for some countries as in Table 6.

and are independent of age in the high-mortality area as well as in Western Europe as a whole.

Female mortality has developed along very different lines and conforms fully to the expected law of diminishing return with advancing age. Prime examples of strong age-selectivity in this direction are Japan, France, Switzerland and all Nordic countries. The tendency is weak in Portugal and Scotland but there is no significant exception to it among the 27 countries examined. The pattern is confirmed in all aggregates.

10.3 Discussion

A satisfactory explanation of the varying age patterns of mortality decline would require an analysis of the causes of death. Some general features observed in the data at hand do, however, permit a few tentative suggestions. As age increases, degenerative diseases such as most heart diseases, arteriosclerosis and the various forms of senile dementia become gradually the prevalent causes of death. Aging itself becomes a prime determinant of mortality. Strong evidence has been published to the effect that wide-spread changes in lifestyle, including diet, smoking and exercise, probably combined with blood pressure control, have been the main factor in reducing mortality from degenerative diseases in industrialized countries. If this is the case and if the aging process itself is delayed, it is natural that its benefits are felt more at ages where it is not yet very advanced. Hence mortality should decline more, say, at age 80 than 90 or 100. Among the still younger elderly, on the other hand, other causes of death with different etiology predominate and even if they depend on lifestyle, they have often been less responsive to recent trends in it.

It appears that in low-mortality societies women live closer to their physical endowment and die more in conformity with the aging process and this results in more regular and more uniform mortality patterns. Men are more prone to death by external events and through morbid processes caused by a multitude of interfering factors. Whether these depend on occupation, lifestyle or other influences, they are more diversified in space and over time and this leads to less uniform mortality patterns. It also follows that findings in studies like the present one are valid only for the kind of populations they represent and in the specified period. They are also liable to change at any time.

11. The case of centenarians

In the earlier chapters little has been shown about ages over 100 years. The numbers have been too small for meaningful period rates or time series for individual countries or even for the aggregates which were formed from them. A still larger grouping is needed.

Reasonably long series of good quality data on centenarian mortality are available in the Odense archive for only thirteen countries of Western Europe. The corresponding data are available also for Japan but the resulting time series is unsteady because in the early decades the numbers were small and possibly inaccurate as would be understandable, birth registration having been introduced only in 1872.

Merged data for the 13 countries are given in Annex Table 8. Smoothed with 5-year moving averages they are illustrated in Figure 6. The results appear to be consistent and credible and allow the conclusion that in the low-mortality zone of Western Europe the mortality of centenarians has been declining throughout the post-war period. There is some evidence of a slowdown from about 1965 to 1975, particularly among men, after which the decline again accelerated.

The death rates for the two sexes have moved in an approximately parallel fashion, the male rate consistently higher than the female, without indicating a tendency to converge as is often claimed to happen. The excess male mortality has fluctuated around 14 - 18 percent without a clear trend.

Another view of centenarian mortality is given in Figure 7 with probabilities of dying at individual ages. It may be pointed out that these probabilities q_x are always lower than central death rates m_x on which Figure 6 was based and that when mortality is high, the difference is quite large. Conceptually, q_x is a more faithful measure of mortality when it is calculated, as in the present study, by following a group of persons from one exact age to the next. When the numbers are small, the greater precision may be important.

In Figure 7 the curves are drawn as far as the number of persons exposed to risk is not less than 100. It can be seen that under this rule the curves extend decade by decade one or two years further up the age scale, testifying to a rapid increase in observed cases. The underlying data are given for 1980-90 in Table 13 and for all decades in Annex Table 9. The very unequal numbers involved may be appreciated from the fact that the 1980-90 curve for females is at age 109 based on only 116 observations but at age 100 on nearly 57,000.

It is evident from Figure 7, first of all, that mortality keeps increasing with advancing age and that there is no sign, at least by age 109, of it approaching a plateau, even less a downturn. Allowing for fluctuations due to small numbers and possible inaccuracies in the earliest data, the curves have retained their ascending form essentially unchanged.

Decennial reductions in mortality can also be observed though they have been rather small until the very substantial drop between the 1970s and 1980s which has been consistent by age for both sexes. The current decline in oldest-old mortality extends to ages over 105 years.

Table 13. PROBABILITY OF DYING AT AGES 100 AND OVER, 1980-1990. Pooled data for 14 countries[1]

Age x	Males			Females		
	Reached age x	Died before age x+1	1000q	Reached age x	Died before age x+1	1000q
100	13 433	5 658	421	56 926	20 927	368
101	7 293	3 097	425	33 003	12 646	383
102	3 856	1 657	430	18 547	7 363	397
103	2 032	942	464	10 249	4 308	420
104	1 007	445	442	5 382	2 332	433
105	495	223	451	2 759	1 267	459
106	243	110	453	1 342	610	455
107	109	53	486	644	307	477
108	53	29		297	167	562
109	19	15		116	70	603
110	5	2		40	21	
111	2	1		14	5	
112				6	2	
113				4	1	
114				3	1	

[1] Austria, Belgium, Denmark, England & Wales, Finland, France, West Germany, Iceland, Italy, Japan, Netherlands, Norway, Sweden and Switzerland.

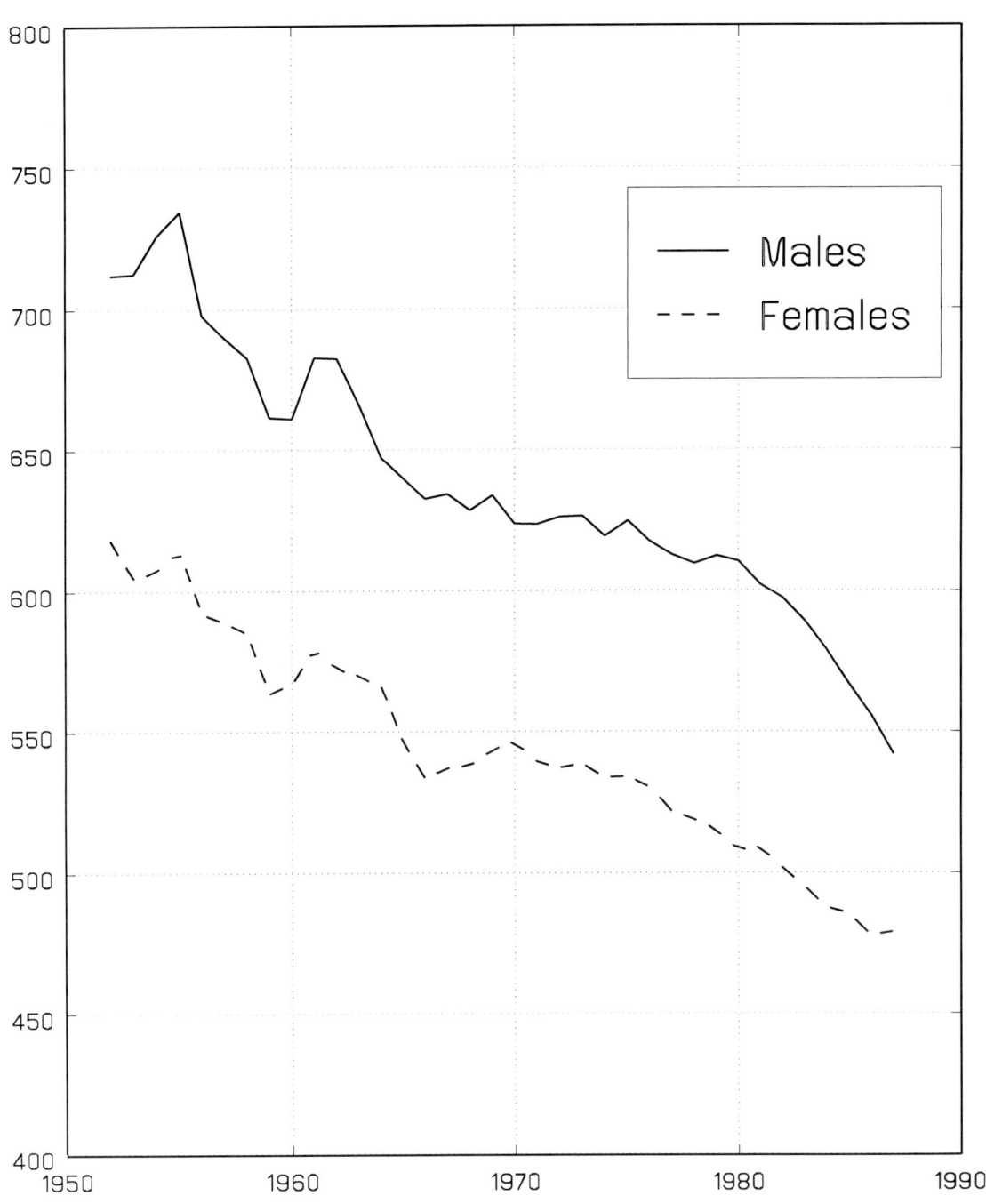

Figure 6. Deaths per 1000 population aged 100 and over in 13 countries of Western Europe
5-year moving averages

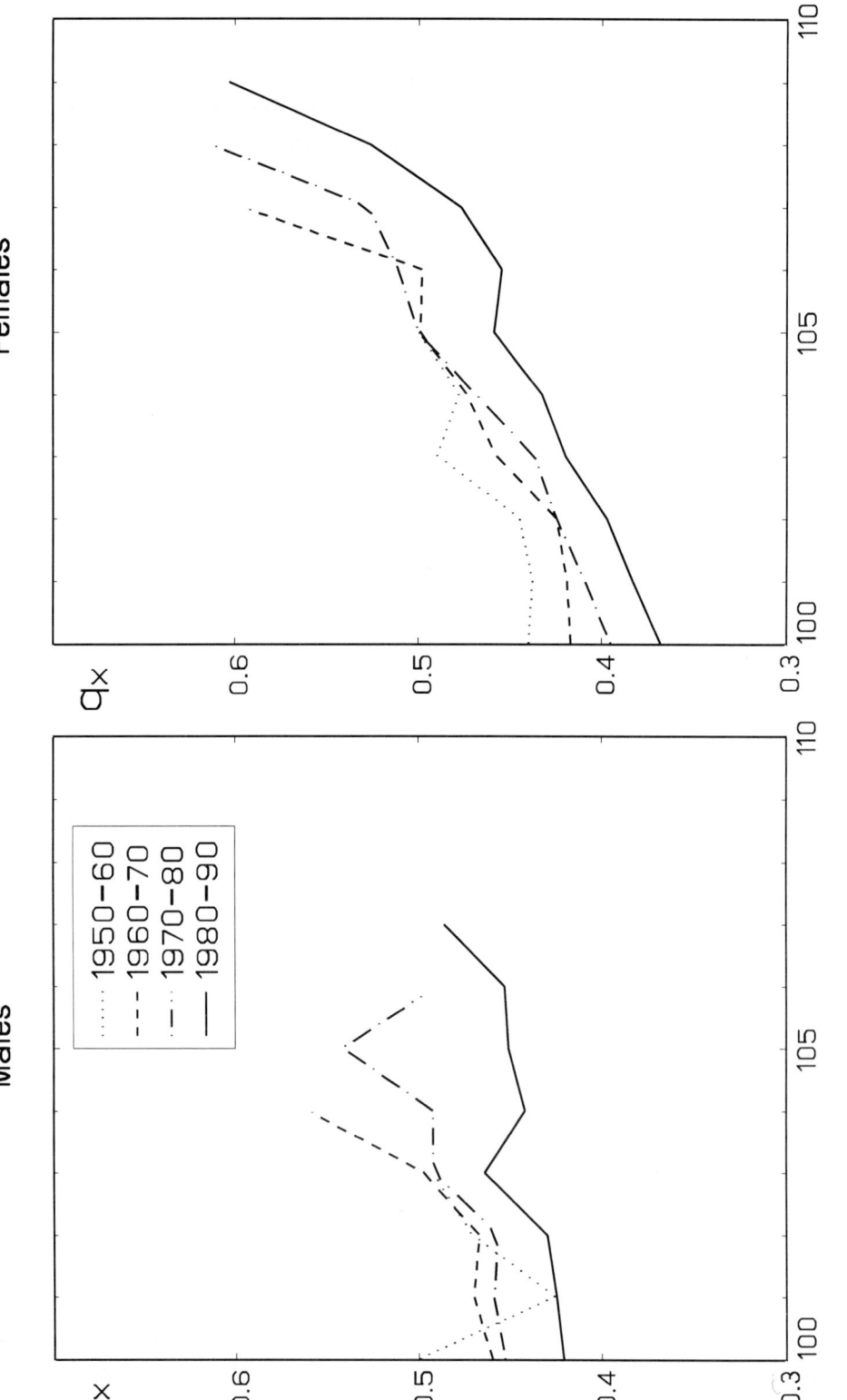

12. Period or cohort effect?

A full analysis of a possible cohort effect in the widespread mortality decline is yet to be made. Instead, the time series in the countries which have been experiencing sudden changes in trend are examined in the following in order to see whether the changes have taken place in different age groups simultaneously or with a time lag which could be indicative of a cohort effect.

The countries in which the sharpest breaks in trend have occurred are Japan, Finland, West Germany, Norway and Czechoslovakia. Instead of annual series which proved too unsteady, we have used quinquennial averages and calculated the percentage change from one to the next. These are shown in Table 14 for the four 5-year age groups below age 100. The development is illustrated in Figure 8 but without the group 95-99 which frequently showed rather erratic values. The following is a commentary of the findings.

Japan

Males. A moderate decline in the 1950s came to a stop around 1960 after which began an ever more precipitous fall. Through all these changes all age groups run parallel though the oldest group only approximately.
Females. A slow initial decline stopped around 1960 after which began a sharp drop simultaneously in all age groups, accelerating till about 1975 after which it has continued apace.

Finland

Males. A slow decline in the 1950s turned into a rise and then, around 1970 into a steep decline which slowed down in the 1980s. All these stages were simultaneous at all ages.
Females. Similar development except that instead of an increase there was a stagnation in the 1960s and the drop after 1970 was even steeper than for men. All changes were closely parallel at all ages.

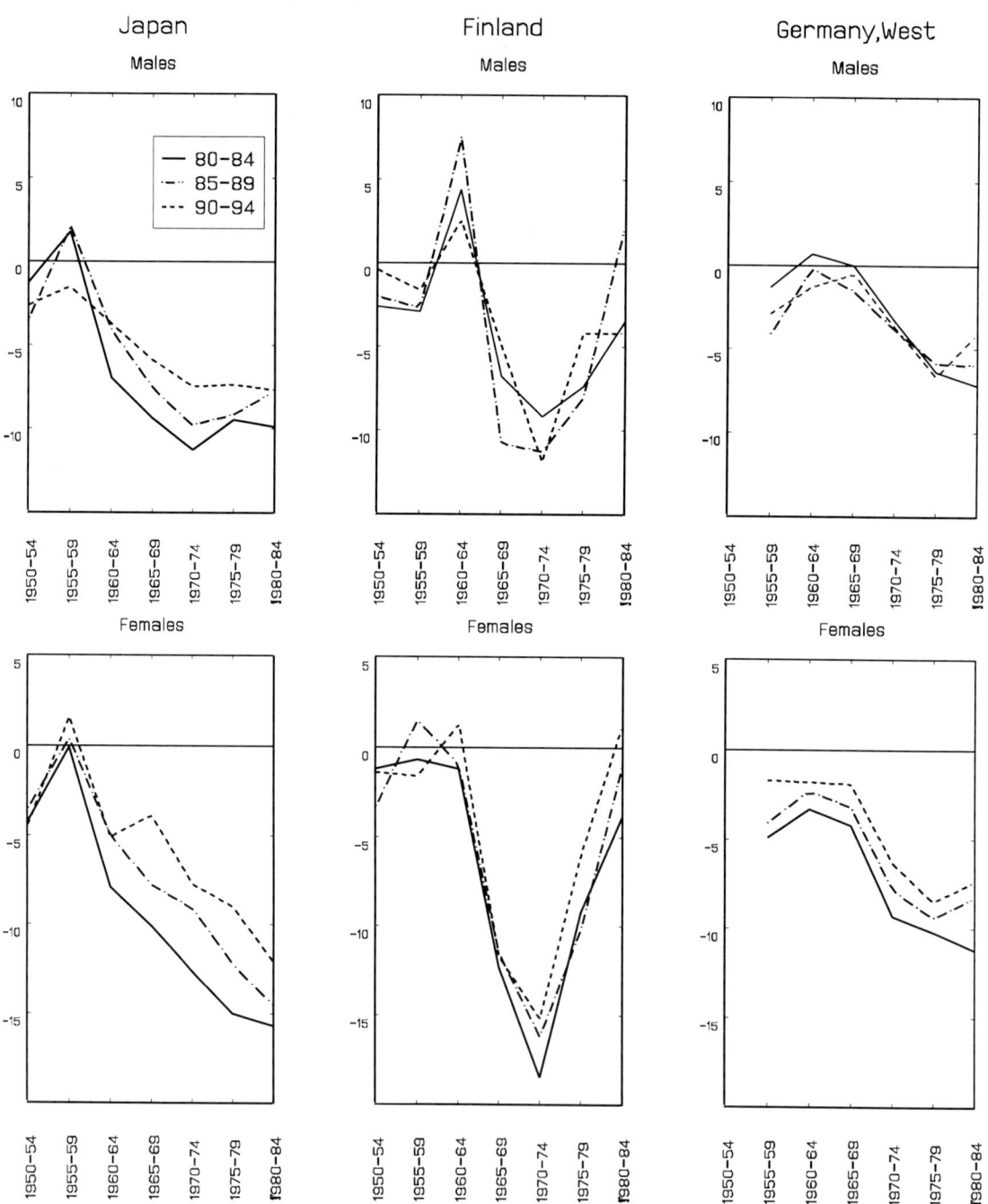

Figure 8. Percent change in age-specific death rate from the given 5-year period to the next.

Figure 8. Percent change in age-specific death rate from the given 5-year period to the next.
(continued)

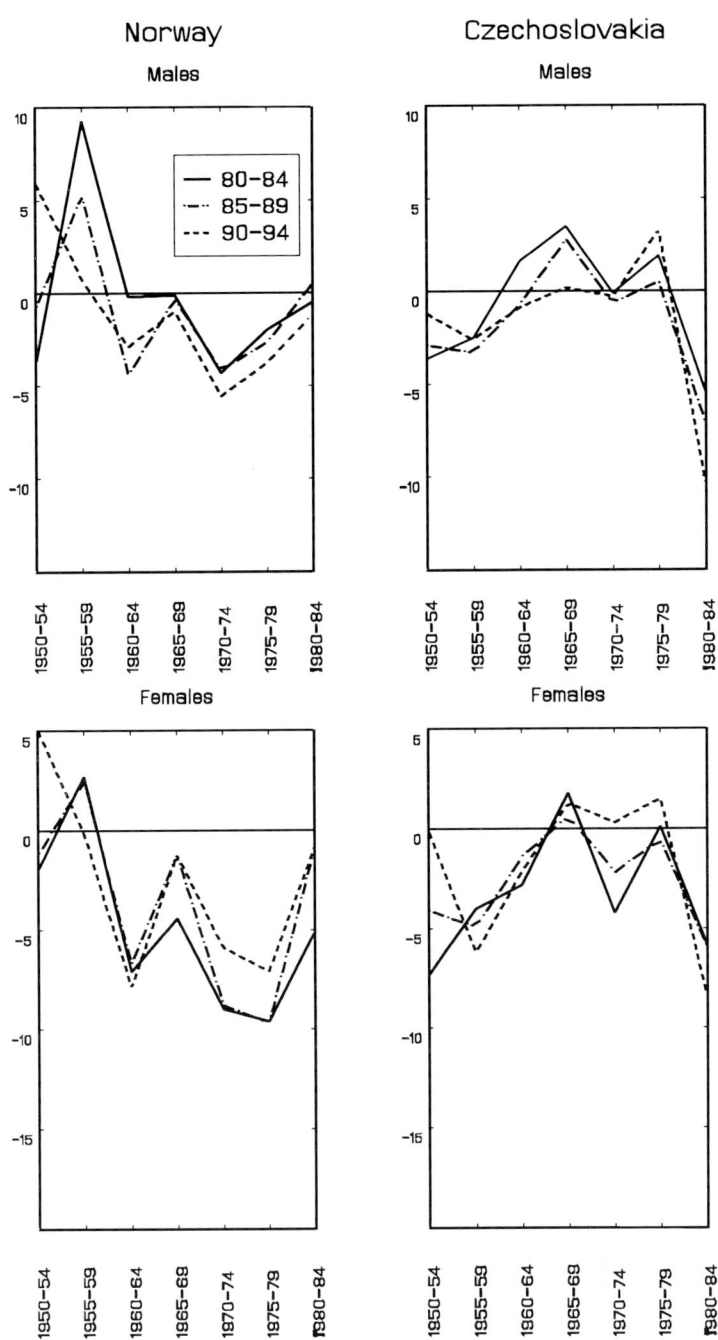

Table 14. PERCENT CHANGE IN AGE-SPECIFIC DEATH RATE FROM GIVEN 5-YEAR PERIOD TO THE NEXT

Country and period	Males				Females			
	80-84	85-89	90-94	95-99	80-84	85-89	90-94	95-99
JAPAN								
1950-54	- 1.2	- 3.4	- 2.6	+ 0.5	- 4.2	- 3.5	- 4.4	+ 4.3
1955-59	+ 1.8	+ 2.1	- 1.5	+ 5.6	- 0.1	+ 0.4	+ 1.6	- 3.0
1960-64	- 7.0	- 4.1	- 3.7	-10.4	- 7.9	- 5.0	- 5.1	- 3.2
1965-69	- 9.4	- 7.6	- 5.9	- 0.7	-10.1	- 7.8	- 3.9	- 4.9
1970-74	-11.3	- 9.8	- 7.5	- 3.9	-12.6	- 9.1	- 7.7	- 4.8
1975-79	- 9.5	- 9.2	- 7.4	- 9.4	-15.0	-12.2	- 9.0	- 6.7
1980-84	- 9.9	- 7.8	- 7.7	- 4.8	-15.7	-14.5	-12.1	- 8.3
FINLAND								
1950-54	- 2.6	- 2.0	- 0.4	...	- 1.2	- 3.3	- 1.4	-16.4
1955-59	- 2.9	- 2.7	- 1.6	...	- 0.7	+ 1.5	- 1.6	+ 3.6
1960-64	+ 4.4	+ 7.5	+ 2.6	...	- 1.2	- 1.0	+ 1.3	+ 3.8
1965-69	- 6.8	-10.8	- 5.0	...	-12.3	-11.5	-11.7	-16.3
1970-74	- 9.2	-11.3	-11.9	...	-18.5	-16.2	-15.2	- 9.8
1975-79	- 7.4	- 8.1	- 4.2	...	- 9.2	-10.2	- 6.0	-13.4
1980-84	- 3.5	+ 2.3	- 4.2	...	- 3.9	- 1.1	+ 1.2	+18.1
GERMANY, W.								
1955-59	- 1.3	- 4.1	- 2.9	+ 4.1	- 4.9	- 4.1	- 1.7	- 1.4
1960-64	+ 0.7	- 0.2	- 1.3	- 3.1	- 3.3	- 2.3	- 1.8	- 1.4
1965-69	-	- 1.5	- 0.5	- 3.5	- 4.2	- 3.2	- 1.9	+ 1.7
1970-74	- 3.3	- 3.8	- 3.7	+ 2.0	- 9.3	- 7.8	- 6.2	- 5.6
1975-79	- 6.4	- 5.9	- 6.7	- 7.3	-10.2	- 9.4	- 8.5	-10.0
1980-84	- 7.2	- 6.0	- 4.1	- 9.1	-11.2	- 8.3	- 7.4	- 9.4
NORWAY								
1950-54	- 3.6	- 0.7	+ 5.9	- 2.5	- 1.9	- 1.1	+ 5.0	- 0.6
1955-59	+ 9.3	+ 5.3	+ 0.7	+ 1.8	+ 2.7	+ 2.5	- 0.2	+ 8.0
1960-64	- 0.2	- 4.4	- 2.9	- 9.1	- 7.1	- 6.7	- 7.9	-10.2
1965-69	- 0.1	- 0.3	- 1.0	- 1.9	- 4.4	- 1.2	- 1.2	- 3.3
1970-74	- 4.3	- 4.2	- 5.6	+ 5.8	- 9.0	- 8.8	- 5.9	- 7.7
1975-79	- 2.0	- 2.7	- 3.8	-12.1	- 9.6	- 9.7	- 7.1	- 4.5
1980-84	- 0.5	+ 0.5	- 1.2	+ 5.9	- 5.2	- 1.0	- 0.9	+ 1.3
CZECHO-SLOVAKIA								
1950-54	- 3.6	- 2.9	- 1.2	- 7.6	- 7.3	- 4.1	- 0.2	- 6.5
1955-59	- 2.5	- 3.3	- 2.6	+13.2	- 4.0	- 4.9	- 6.2	- 4.1
1960-64	+ 1.6	- 0.7	- 0.9	- 4.7	- 2.8	- 1.4	- 2.1	- 2.3
1965-69	+ 3.5	+ 2.8	+ 0.2	-10.9	+ 1.8	+ 0.6	+ 1.3	- 1.1
1970-74	- 0.1	- 0.7	- 0.3	- 0.8	- 4.2	- 2.2	+ 0.3	- 1.0
1975-79	+ 1.9	+ 0.5	+ 3.3	+ 9.0	+ 0.1	- 0.6	+ 1.5	+ 5.3
1980-84	- 5.4	- 7.1	-10.3	+ 2.7	- 5.8	- 5.9	- 8.4	- 2.3

West Germany

After a slow improvement during the first two decades, a sharp fall began simultaneously for both sexes and all age groups around 1975 and it has continued until now.

Norway

Sharp drops have alternated with relative slowdowns and even an increase around 1960, always simultaneously for both sexes and all ages though with always a more favourable development for females.

Czechoslovakia

Males. Initial improvement which may be seen as return to normal after the war, was followed by an increase in mortality until the last quinquennium brought about a sudden decline at all ages.
Females. The early improvement was more pronounced and lasted longer than with men. It was followed by a period of approximate stagnation and finally a sharp drop, similarly at all ages.

To sum up, the development in any given country and for each sex has been closely simultaneous in all age groups, particularly the three younger ones which display the steadiest rates. Every important change in trend, whether up or down, has taken place virtually at the same time at all ages without any indication of time lag at older ages. It may be noted in particular that the time of onset of a rapid mortality decline has been simultaneous in the different age groups and therefore has not been produced gradually by supposedly healthier cohorts moving into higher ages. The existence of cohort factors is not precluded but it is obvious that their role, if any, has been only secondary and that the recent epoch-making decline in old age mortality has been caused by period factors with immediate effect.

13. Sex ratio and sex differential of mortality

The greater longevity of the human female is most clearly manifest in the life of the elderly and translates virtually without exception into a sex ratio of mortality (male rate per female rate) higher than unity. With increasing age, however, this ratio - likewise almost universally - declines and this has often led to the mistaken conclusion that at high ages death rates for the two sexes tend to converge and may eventually intersect.

Actually, the declining ratio is nothing more than an inevitable result of arithmetic: at young ages the ratio may reach, and often does, values of 2 or 3 but such ratios become increasingly unlikely and finally impossible as mortality reaches higher levels in old age. If, instead of the ratio, we look at the differential of the rates, the picture changes completely: instead of converging, the rates maintain their distance.

These two structural features of old age mortality - sex ratio declining but sex differential fairly constant with advancing age - have persisted through the recent momentous development which has been much more beneficial to women than men.

An examination of the sex ratio based on age-standardized death rates at ages 80-99 in the 28 countries with acceptable data (Annex Table 10) confirms, first of all, that the males are subject to considerably higher mortality than the females and that this difference has lately been increasing. The male excess mortality which at these ages in 1960-64 varied between countries from 10 to 33 percent, had by 1985-89 grown to an excess of 24 to 48 percent while the mean had grown from 20 to 36 percent.

The highest levels of excess male mortality in old age are now found in Northwestern Europe and Australia as shown in Table 15 and the lowest generally in Eastern and Central Europe. The very low ratio for Spain is probably due to age overstatement by males whose death rate therefore has a downward bias.

The increase in the sex ratio during this last quarter century, also shown in Table 15, has been remarkably sharp in the Low Countries and Scandinavia where improvement in the mortality of old men has been slight. Although this has not been the case in Switzerland and Finland, the gains were in these countries much larger for women. At the other extreme, the sex ratio has increased only moderately in the former East bloc. The apparent decline in Spain is most likely an artifact. The development is illustrated by age group in Figure 9 which is composed of only the most reliable data. In it an aggregate of eleven Western European countries is compared with a group of three Eastern European countries and with Japan. The actual ratios are given in Annex Table 11.

In both European groups the decline of the sex ratio of mortality with advancing age was very moderate in the 1950s, after which the gradually increasing female advantage has translated into ever steeper slopes as the upper end of the life span has not kept pace with the rapid changes among octogenarians. In Japan the slope was very straight and stable for three decades and approached the European pattern only in the 1980s when it also confirmed the existence of a mortality difference between male and female centenarians.

Table 15.   SEX RATIO OF MORTALITY AT AGES 80-99 YEARS.

1985-89		Increase from 1960-64	
Netherlands	1.480	Netherlands	0.357
England & Wales	1.473	Luxemburg	0.293
Scotland	1.463	Sweden	0.292
Australia	1.450	Denmark	0.281
Luxemburg	1.450	Norway	0.271
France	1.446	Switzerland	0.250
Sweden	1.434	Finland	0.243
Switzerland	1.426	Germany, West	0.223
Denmark	1.408	Belgium	0.214
Belgium	1.407	Italy	0.178
Japan	1.404	Scotland	0.175
New Zealand	1.398	Ireland	0.167
Norway	1.396	Iceland	0.166
Germany, West	1.376	Japan	0.157
Ireland	1.373	France	0.152
Italy	1.346	England & Wales	0.150
Finland	1.338	Germany, East	0.143
Iceland	1.323	New Zealand	0.122
Singapore	1.299	Hungary	0.121
Portugal	1.294	Australia	0.118
Estonia	1.280	Czechoslovakia	0.091
Germany, East	1.265	Latvia	0.072
Hungary	1.265	Austria	0.051
Austria	1.263	Estonia	0.039
Czechoslovakia	1.259	Portugal	0.024
Poland	1.259	Spain	- 0.008
Latvia	1.256	Singapore	...
Spain	1.237	Poland	...
Mean of 28	1.360	Mean of 26	0.167

Figure 9. Sex ratio of mortality

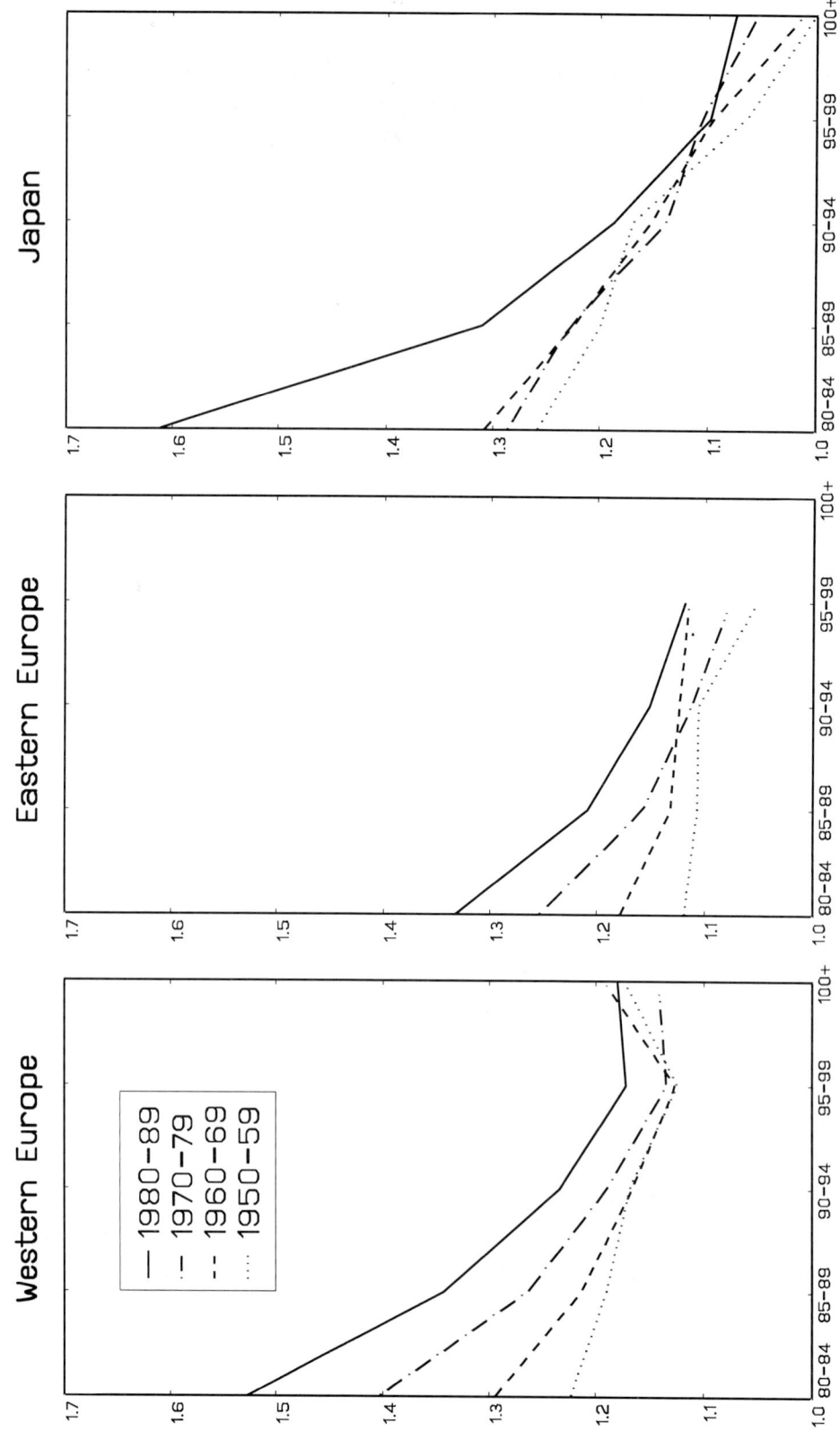

When, instead of sex ratio, we look at the sex differential in Figure 10, we note its nearly constant size by age. In the European curves there is a tendency for a slow increase of the differential over age which belies the assumption of convergence. As the female advantage has grown over time, the curves have been moving to higher levels while roughly maintaining their slowly ascending form.

14. Effect of differential mortality on population sex ratio

In view of the development which has been markedly more favourable for the survival of females than males (and not only at old age), one would expect a commensurate and sustained increase in the proportion of women in old age populations as well. While such an increase has certainly taken place, it has not been entirely universal and has largely come to a stop or even turned into a decrease in the 1980s.

Figure 11 shows the development of the sex ratio among the oldest-old population in 28 countries. Because of the lopsided relation in favour of women, it was found more illuminative to invert the usual sex ratio and give the number of women per men.

In five countries (Iceland, Japan, Poland, Portugal and Spain) the sex ratio did not change much during the period observed. In the other 23, the ratio of females per male increased rapidly during most of the period and the excess of females over males doubled or tripled in many cases. In the 1980s, however, a drastic change took place: in 8 countries (including England & Wales, France and Australia), the ratio turned decisively down while in 6 others it stopped growing. It continued to increase in 9 countries but in some of them at slower speed.

The explanation of the paradox of a growing proportion of men in the population while the mortality of women was declining faster, lies not in the death rates but in the numbers of lives saved. Because male mortality is higher than the female, a proportionate decline in both and even a somewhat smaller decline in the former, results in the saving of more male than female lives. As these are cumulated age by age, the number of men reaching an advanced age will grow relatively faster than that of women reaching the same age. Fluctuations in sex ratio are also caused by the succession of male cohorts, some of which have suffered war losses and others not.

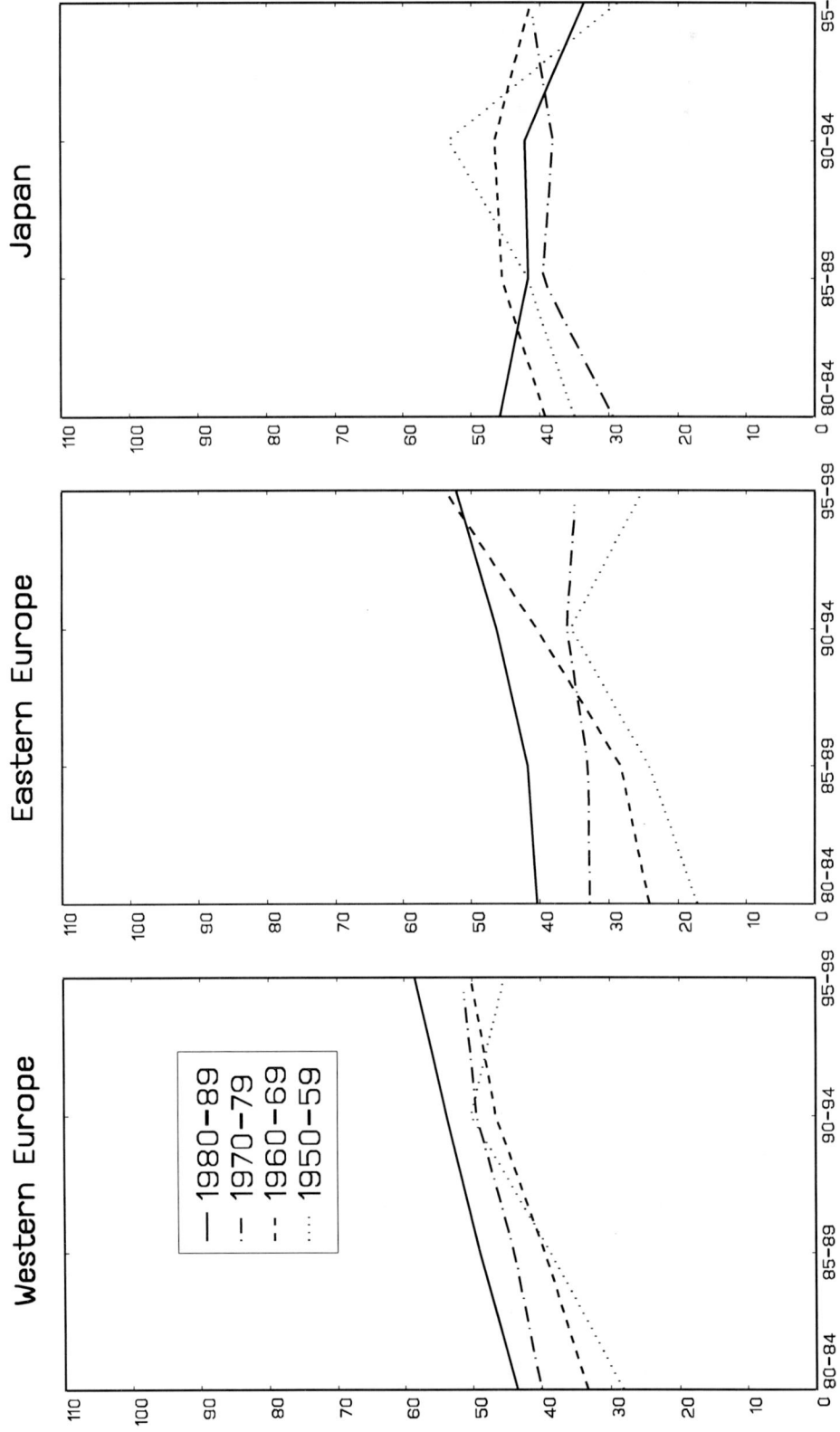

Figure 10. Sex differential of mortality per 1000 population

Figure 11. Sex ratio of population aged 80 and over

F/M

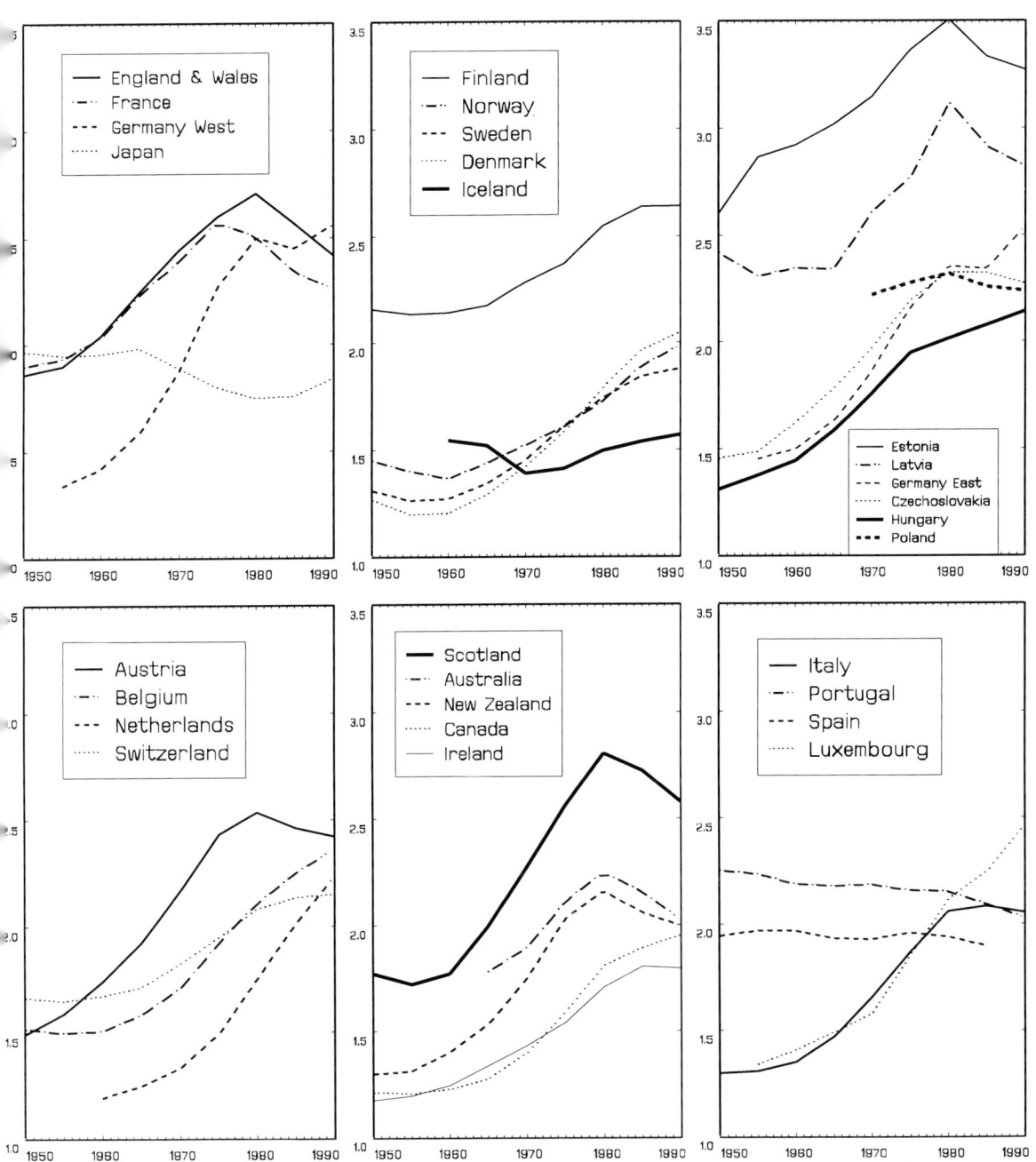

Another way to understand the process is to consider that more boys are born than girls, the excess being about 5 percent. In the past, this excess was wiped out in a few years so that at the latest when the cohort reached marriageable age, the numbers of both sexes were equal, and after that, women outnumbered men. This is no longer happening. Premature mortality is in developed countries now so low that although it still is higher for males than females, parity in numbers is reached only around age 50 or even later. Consequently, among those reaching an advanced age, the proportion of males has begun to increase. In numerous countries of the database this has happened in the 1980s to persons reaching age 80. The same, however, is not yet happening to those reaching age 90 or 100.

15. Conclusions

Death rates at ages 80 and over have been calculated for the post-1950 period for 28 low-mortality countries that process sufficiently reliable data on deaths by single years of age to allow the use of the extinct cohorts method. The material available covers most of the countries representative of the low-mortality countries of the world.

The study shows that mortality in old age has undergone in the developed countries during the post-war period a deep-going and fairly general transformation reaching much lower levels than have ever been recorded before. Unprecedented in known demographic history, this decline has made in the prevailing trend a break which had not been foreseen in population projections.

The new wave of mortality decline has varied from country to country as to its onset as well as to rapidity and extent and has in some been interrupted by periods of stagnation or temporary increase. The age pattern of decline has varied from an essentially uniform one to one favouring either the relatively younger or the very oldest. The decline has reached the highest ages in which mortality can today be empirically measured, i.e. ages of 107-109 years.

Among the great variety of national situations there has been on the whole a perceptible tendency of the decline to accelerate in more recent years. Yet, the development has not been leading towards convergence between countries, on the contrary. The only feature common to all 28 countries observed has been a development more favourable to the survival of women than of men, thus widening the already existing female advantage.

Looking for the causes of this development we should note first of all that during the post-war period increasing numbers of persons have been reaching the age 80, the starting line of observation in the present study. The reasons for this increase lie partly in the past as advances in medicine and in living conditions have permitted people to reach higher ages. At the same time and perhaps because of it, old persons are receiving increased medical attention.

While all this has created a long-term trend for improved survival, we have seen in the present study that important factors have come into play after 1950 and particularly in the last decades, reducing mortality even at the oldest ages in an unprecedented manner. These reductions have in most cases been comparable to and simultaneous with reductions in mortality among the younger elderly.

These new factors which are distinctively period rather than cohort factors may include further advances in medical practice such as more generalized control of blood pressure but there is on the other hand solid evidence from many countries to the effect that an important and probably the main factor has been a change for a healthier lifestyle - a change which has been shown to have almost immediate effects on the probability of survival. Such behavioural changes prevent or delay the onset of morbid processes which would in time lead to serious health impairment or death. Maybe the aging process itself is thereby delayed.

Studies from various countries have shown that the new lifestyle has been adopted first by the better educated, wealthy, urban sectors of the population and has been gradually filtering through to other social strata. The time lag in this process has almost certainly contributed to creating or aggravating social differentials in mortality which have been observed in many large-scale studies.

The novelty and magnitude of the observed mortality decline seem to justify it being called *a new stage in mortality transition*. In contrast to the earlier stages in which the main benefits accrued to childhood and working age, the new stage is characterized by mortality decline in later life where the main beneficiaries are the elderly from their sixties to the eighties and nineties and, to a hardly lesser extent, even beyond.

We do not, as yet, know the ultimate extent of the new mortality transition. But considering that the new lifestyle has not yet been anything like universally adopted, a vast potential exists for further improvement in health. And since this social process seems to be going on and as there is at the present time a strong downward momentum in death rates, the new transition may, barring unforeseen events, still continue for an extended period.

Sources

Official statistics on deaths and on population:
Australia. Australian Bureau of Statistics, Belconnen, ACT.
Austria. Oesterreichisches Statistisches Zentralamt, Wien.
Belgium. Institut National de Statistique, Bruxelles.
Canada. Statistics Canada, Ottawa.
Chile. Instituto Nacional de Estadistica, Santiago.
Czechoslovakia. Federal Statistical Office, Praha.
Denmark. Danmarks Statistik, Copenhagen.
England and Wales. Office of Population Censuses and Surveys, London.
Estonia. Eesti Demograafia Assotsiatsioon, Tallinn.
Finland. Tilastokeskus, Helsinki.
France. Institut National de la Statistique et des Etudes Economiques, Paris.
Germany, East. Gemeinsames Statistisches Amt, Berlin.
Germany, West. Statistisches Bundesamt, Wiesbaden.
Hungary. Central Statistical Office, Budapest.
Iceland. Hagstofa Islands, Reykjavik.
Ireland. Central Statistics Office, Dublin.
Italy. Instituto Nazionale di Statistica, Roma.
Japan. Deaths: Statistics and Information Department, Ministry of Health and Welfare, Tokyo. Population: Statistics Bureau, Management and Coordination Agency, Tokyo.
Latvia. Department of Statistics and Demography, Faculty of Economics, University of Riga.
Luxemburg. Service Central de Statistique et des Etudes Economiques, Luxemburg.
Netherlands. Centraal Bureau voor de Statistiek, Voorburg.
New Zealand. Department of Statistics, Christchurch.
Norway. Statistisk Sentralbyra, Oslo.
Poland. Central Statistical Office, Warszawa.
Portugal. Instituto Nacional de Estadistica, Lisboa.
Scotland. General Register Office for Scotland, Edinburgh.
Singapore. Department of Statistics, Singapore.
Spain. Instituto Nacional de Estadistica, Madrid.
Sweden. Statistics Sweden, Stockholm.
Switzerland. Bundesamt für Statistik, Bern.
United Nations. Statistical Division, New York.
United States. National Center for Health Statistics, Hyattsville, Maryland.

References

VINCENT, Paul (1951), La Mortalité des vieillards. Population, 6 (2): 181-204. Paris.
DEPOID, Françoise (1973), La Mortalité des grands vieillards. Population 28: 755-792. Paris.
KANNISTO, Väinö (1990), Mortality of the elderly in late 19th and early 20th century Finland. Tilastokeskus, Studies 175. 49 pp. Helsinki.

Annex Tables
Vaïnö Kannisto, Jens Lauritsen, Kirill Andreev

1. Persons and deaths in 1950-1990 in the Kannisto-Thatcher Oldest-Old Database.
2. Age-standardized death rates at ages 80 - 99 in 1950-1990. 28 countries.
3. Age-standardized death rates at ages 80 - 99 by 5-year periods in 1950-1989. 28 countries.
4. Age-standardized death rates at ages 80 - 99 in 1950-1990. Selected groups of countries.
5. Age-standardized death rates at ages 80-99. Average of last five annual rates. Male/Female
6. Mortality of the elderly in 1955-59 and 1985-89 by age and sex. Selected countries.
7. Death rates by age and sex in 1950 - 1989. Groups of countries.
8. Deaths per 1000 population aged 100 and over in 1950 - 1989 in Western Europe.
9. Probability of dying at ages 100 and over by decade.
10. Sex ratio of mortality at ages 80 - 99, by country.
11. Sex ratio of mortality by age by groups of countries.
12. Standard population: Sweden, both sexes, 1950-1989.

ANNEX TABLE 1. PERSONS AND DEATHS IN 1950-1990 IN THE KANNISTO-THATCHER OLDEST-OLD DATABASE

Country	Persons			Deaths		
	Total	Male	Female	Total	Male	Female
Australia	1 197 897	445 135	752 762	816 253	318 250	498 003
Austria	1 394 555	479 506	915 049	1 096 956	392 016	704 940
Belgium	1 771 296	666 659	1 104 637	1 403 551	558 504	845 047
Canada	2 210 632	942 877	1 267 755	1 606 460	738 846	867 614
Chile	253 871	96 084	157 787	137 632	56 301	81 331
Czechoslovakia	1 855 484	667 683	1 187 801	1 487 927	555 092	932 835
Denmark	817 445	336 709	480 736	625 012	273 589	351 423
England and Wales	8 804 705	3 023 415	5 781 290	6 888 902	2 457 860	4 431 042
Estonia	216 292	57 750	158 542	174 444	48 126	126 318
Finland	547 141	174 614	372 527	403 595	135 285	268 310
France	9 514 765	3 302 570	6 212 195	7 310 256	2 619 595	4 690 661
Germany,East	3 181 850	1 117 155	2 064 695	2 614 022	963 932	1 650 090
Germany,West	10 498 512	3 690 649	6 807 863	7 932 494	2 984 417	4 948 077
Hungary	1 394 921	529 750	865 171	1 126 013	444 668	681 345
Iceland	21 151	9 006	12 145	14 830	6 545	8 285
Ireland	473 787	207 039	266 748	396 552	179 404	217 148
Italy	7 501 380	2 933 565	4 567 815	5 755 867	2 362 350	3 393 517
Japan	10 042 347	3 888 501	6 153 846	6 919 610	2 811 231	4 108 379
Latvia	373 102	111 195	261 907	298 497	91 847	206 650
Luxemburg	49 562	18 809	30 753	38 147	15 516	22 631
Netherlands	1 514 599	609 185	905 414	1 085 271	476 430	608 841
Norway	670 036	271 045	398 991	513 755	218 653	295 102
New Zealand,Maori	4 307	2 156	2 151	3 805	1 949	1 856
New Zealand,Non Maori	331 558	132 336	199 222	257 204	107 710	149 494
Poland	2 356 897	791 970	1 564 927	1 589 993	555 834	1 034 159
Portugal	1 203 120	426 215	776 905	948 852	341 847	607 005
Scotland	875 854	302 972	572 882	699 925	253 503	446 422
Singapore,Chinese	49 249	18 232	31 017	22 043	8 440	13 603
Spain	3 710 765	1 378 202	2 332 563	2 746 367	1 044 437	1 701 930
Sweden	1 479 188	618 866	860 322	1 120 253	494 092	626 161
Switzerland	996 263	371 096	625 167	736 200	288 730	447 470
Total	75 312 531	27 620 946	47 691 585	56 770 688	21 804 999	34 965 689

ANNEX TABLE 2. AGE-STANDARDIZED DEATH RATES AT AGES 80-99.
MALE

Year	Australia	Austria	Belgium	Czecho-slovakia	Denmark	England & Wales	Estonia
1950	...	200.7	200.4	204.5	189.6	207.5	225.3
1951	...	213.1	207.6	212.3	169.6	224.3	214.7
1952	...	208.1	199.4	211.3	174.8	201.7	242.6
1953	...	206.3	203.8	223.7	178.5	199.4	219.0
1954	...	208.6	195.7	219.0	177.0	201.3	205.9
1955	...	206.9	207.1	198.2	168.6	208.2	198.1
1956	...	208.9	199.6	205.0	169.2	206.6	174.7
1957	...	200.4	191.3	216.4	175.0	191.7	187.8
1958	...	196.6	187.4	205.2	178.0	200.6	189.2
1959	...	196.6	183.6	212.2	171.1	194.3	195.8
1960	...	204.6	198.2	201.2	177.4	188.8	182.7
1961	...	188.9	184.1	195.4	172.1	195.7	202.2
1962	...	205.4	193.3	223.2	178.4	198.2	205.4
1963	...	204.1	202.7	198.3	176.9	204.3	192.6
1964	...	188.4	178.9	194.8	175.8	179.3	163.1
1965	173.1	200.9	184.7	201.1	175.2	183.8	193.1
1966	181.6	190.1	184.8	200.9	182.5	189.7	186.4
1967	171.0	200.3	184.9	200.0	164.7	176.6	180.7
1968	190.8	199.9	198.8	209.4	163.6	191.5	179.1
1969	170.1	196.7	190.8	204.8	160.7	180.9	181.6
1970	180.5	200.9	183.1	209.0	154.2	179.5	180.7
1971	175.6	200.6	187.1	209.3	159.2	178.0	180.2
1972	172.8	194.0	182.6	200.0	152.3	185.0	187.8
1973	170.3	189.7	189.1	210.7	155.5	182.8	187.0
1974	182.1	192.3	183.0	211.3	158.9	182.0	180.5
1975	164.9	201.0	192.5	210.6	152.6	181.6	179.8
1976	172.9	195.5	189.8	208.5	162.3	187.1	192.0
1977	158.5	187.3	171.5	209.1	144.6	174.5	166.7
1978	156.9	196.1	176.0	203.8	150.4	175.6	192.2
1979	149.7	185.5	173.4	205.0	158.4	177.7	195.9
1980	150.9	185.6	175.3	220.1	156.0	172.4	188.4
1981	150.4	188.4	172.9	208.0	157.3	170.8	187.5
1982	155.9	180.3	169.1	209.7	150.0	170.9	176.1
1983	145.2	181.8	178.4	212.7	153.6	168.5	174.6
1984	141.2	170.2	167.9	205.6	151.7	161.4	181.0
1985	152.7	175.7	169.6	203.5	153.4	169.6	187.3
1986	138.9	167.6	172.3	207.2	147.1	162.8	179.5
1987	140.7	158.5	156.5	191.4	147.9	154.0	181.1
1988	138.8	155.6	154.9	190.2	150.1	153.5	178.5
1989	145.0	154.1	161.7	196.1	146.2	156.4	171.1
1990	132.3	147.9	156.8	192.4	152.4	153.2	178.5

ANNEX TABLE 2 (cont.)
MALE

Year	Finland	France	Germany East	Germany West	Hungary	Iceland	Ireland
1950	211.4	203.5	...	...	189.7	...	207.0
1951	213.9	220.2	...	...	223.5	...	226.6
1952	216.7	200.2	...	...	228.5	...	181.1
1953	220.5	216.5	...	...	246.8	...	179.4
1954	210.0	197.5	207.9	...	218.7	...	190.3
1955	220.4	200.9	194.3	...	195.3	...	206.3
1956	207.9	211.1	196.9	196.1	202.9	...	180.9
1957	216.5	198.8	202.6	199.6	208.2	...	184.3
1958	202.6	188.2	197.4	192.7	188.7	...	191.8
1959	197.3	186.2	203.8	190.2	207.5	...	190.8
1960	200.0	192.9	211.1	201.7	208.0	...	182.9
1961	195.3	179.1	200.1	186.1	191.5	147.0	198.5
1962	217.9	196.9	217.4	193.4	231.2	143.8	196.9
1963	204.7	196.6	193.6	201.5	191.4	163.0	190.1
1964	203.3	176.8	197.4	178.5	192.9	165.3	182.3
1965	218.3	185.2	209.7	190.2	213.6	142.5	185.6
1966	210.2	172.1	196.2	188.6	185.0	153.9	203.7
1967	209.7	178.3	199.4	185.8	195.0	154.5	171.3
1968	215.4	180.9	216.7	202.5	212.2	147.4	186.3
1969	214.8	179.9	213.1	194.4	203.8	151.6	188.0
1970	204.3	171.2	202.3	191.0	206.3	141.0	184.0
1971	203.5	174.0	202.4	192.9	200.7	155.8	170.2
1972	196.7	166.3	200.1	190.3	197.7	151.0	187.8
1973	187.3	172.7	202.8	192.6	204.4	145.6	189.4
1974	194.9	167.3	198.6	188.6	195.8	131.7	194.0
1975	185.6	170.2	210.6	194.8	202.8	129.8	178.2
1976	184.8	179.5	205.4	189.2	203.5	112.7	190.6
1977	178.8	159.6	195.3	179.0	197.2	124.1	190.8
1978	174.4	164.7	202.2	183.4	207.4	111.5	186.0
1979	166.2	159.5	206.7	176.5	195.4	131.4	188.5
1980	177.7	160.3	211.7	175.6	211.1	132.3	186.9
1981	166.0	162.8	207.3	177.3	200.5	136.9	182.1
1982	156.6	155.4	204.1	172.4	204.2	125.4	180.7
1983	167.6	160.1	201.1	173.8	205.7	133.4	180.5
1984	157.2	152.3	201.1	165.7	203.1	108.7	176.3
1985	176.5	156.7	209.6	168.0	207.1	125.0	183.0
1986	157.5	151.3	206.5	165.2	200.0	116.3	185.9
1987	159.6	144.0	196.1	159.7	192.7	130.5	168.9
1988	159.4	139.6	196.4	156.9	187.8	125.7	166.4
1989	156.2	138.2	189.9	159.1	191.2	129.6	168.3
1990	161.6	136.6	189.0	159.4	191.3	...	...

ANNEX TABLE 2 (cont.)
MALE

Year	Italy	Japan	Latvia	Luxem-burg	Nether-lands	New Zealand	Norway
1950	...	225.6	188.7	...	...	173.8	168.0
1951	...	210.3	191.1	...	...	173.7	149.8
1952	177.6	203.5	181.5	...	...	168.7	153.0
1953	172.6	230.3	189.6	231.4	...	157.1	154.4
1954	150.6	200.6	185.2	190.5	...	166.0	151.5
1955	169.9	196.1	179.1	196.3	...	156.2	149.9
1956	200.0	217.0	172.0	221.6	...	174.6	154.1
1957	180.3	231.8	173.6	222.0	...	175.1	153.0
1958	168.6	199.4	160.2	206.0	...	160.7	155.4
1959	164.5	203.9	176.7	199.4	...	175.4	154.7
1960	178.2	217.1	162.8	221.7	166.5	167.1	160.1
1961	168.6	215.9	166.6	198.4	159.0	164.2	162.2
1962	185.2	227.4	177.9	241.0	171.9	179.6	162.7
1963	185.6	201.8	170.8	189.8	171.4	175.4	171.9
1964	171.7	202.5	157.4	167.2	150.3	180.6	159.2
1965	185.9	217.2	164.6	215.5	160.7	169.5	157.6
1966	178.9	196.5	161.6	193.3	159.4	177.9	162.6
1967	183.9	196.9	165.6	199.3	149.7	160.3	156.5
1968	198.3	199.7	167.3	175.8	162.8	183.0	159.1
1969	189.6	193.4	165.9	190.3	157.3	176.4	161.4
1970	170.8	193.3	171.6	201.4	157.9	173.4	160.3
1971	171.4	183.2	159.9	200.5	158.2	173.2	159.5
1972	166.2	178.3	163.3	192.8	161.6	170.3	159.5
1973	179.9	185.7	172.5	197.6	156.3	170.8	160.2
1974	172.4	182.1	158.6	198.0	149.9	172.4	154.7
1975	178.7	176.2	175.6	180.3	160.2	170.6	155.7
1976	177.4	175.5	174.1	219.1	158.8	172.5	154.9
1977	175.7	163.6	171.4	194.2	144.7	172.3	149.5
1978	170.9	161.5	173.1	195.9	152.3	152.7	151.0
1979	169.0	153.1	175.7	175.6	145.8	158.8	150.5
1980	173.4	160.5	171.5	183.6	148.0	177.7	147.8
1981	168.4	154.6	169.7	190.6	149.5	155.3	153.9
1982	159.9	145.5	160.4	174.6	149.1	158.9	145.6
1983	169.2	148.8	167.7	185.4	148.9	154.9	145.7
1984	155.9	144.3	171.5	172.2	148.7	152.2	147.1
1985	159.0	143.3	184.4	179.1	152.1	163.3	149.5
1986	156.6	137.8	170.6	186.6	152.1	156.4	145.1
1987	149.0	133.8	171.9	176.7	146.9	156.1	149.4
1988	150.5	138.8	179.0	166.2	148.1	153.6	147.4
1989	146.1	134.5	167.8	169.9	154.2	149.5	147.9
1990	...	135.1	182.1	...	...	140.7	...

ANNEX TABLE 2 (cont.)
MALE

Year	Poland	Portugal	Scotland	Singapore	Spain	Sweden	Switzerland
1950	...	192.6	222.4	...	186.9	189.4	188.2
1951	...	207.3	234.8	...	209.4	191.0	207.7
1952	...	191.2	219.0	...	174.6	181.0	193.5
1953	...	201.3	200.8	...	185.7	178.0	202.4
1954	...	201.5	217.8	...	177.9	174.7	194.4
1955	...	201.0	214.0	...	182.3	171.3	198.8
1956	...	242.4	212.8	...	206.0	175.8	202.5
1957	...	207.3	205.8	...	197.9	181.1	192.4
1958	...	184.3	209.7	...	174.8	174.2	178.8
1959	...	202.4	208.0	...	178.6	172.0	180.3
1960	...	205.0	199.5	...	182.7	177.4	187.3
1961	...	194.1	213.5	...	169.2	170.2	173.2
1962	...	196.0	205.9	...	184.7	177.5	190.7
1963	...	211.4	217.6	...	182.8	176.9	197.7
1964	...	193.0	191.5	...	178.2	168.4	179.1
1965	...	198.4	199.1	...	171.6	171.3	186.5
1966	...	207.0	204.5	...	171.1	167.0	180.8
1967	...	196.5	182.1	...	170.5	164.7	171.0
1968	...	193.8	190.4	...	174.0	169.7	183.2
1969	...	211.3	195.4	...	177.8	166.6	177.5
1970	...	189.7	191.8	...	167.9	155.6	173.4
1971	191.7	200.7	182.2	...	183.3	159.9	174.6
1972	173.5	185.4	199.9	...	166.9	157.8	166.1
1973	177.5	194.9	193.6	...	175.1	162.4	164.4
1974	172.2	199.6	194.2	...	170.1	161.3	164.6
1975	179.0	188.5	190.8	...	168.0	162.2	161.1
1976	180.0	197.7	196.7	...	163.8	165.6	165.2
1977	177.9	188.3	182.4	...	159.9	158.8	152.9
1978	184.7	184.3	188.3	...	156.8	157.8	158.2
1979	177.2	175.0	190.5	...	148.8	158.6	155.2
1980	190.2	179.3	186.2	...	148.1	159.2	157.3
1981	174.2	176.5	184.9	...	146.3	157.4	156.7
1982	172.3	166.6	186.2	149.1	139.2	152.5	150.8
1983	178.0	174.2	181.4	160.7	145.4	153.5	155.3
1984	186.0	176.6	173.2	150.2	138.9	147.2	145.4
1985	195.8	177.2	175.8	137.9	144.2	154.6	147.1
1986	188.6	169.1	179.5	134.1	137.3	149.9	143.4
1987	186.3	164.6	170.1	126.1	...	148.6	138.5
1988	178.9	174.1	167.9	136.2	...	152.9	141.3
1989	180.4	167.6	179.7	126.0	...	141.3	141.2
1990	180.7	181.7	163.6	119.3	...	144.9	146.1

ANNEX TABLE 2 (cont.)
FEMALE

Year	Australia	Austria	Belgium	Czecho-slovakia	Denmark	England & Wales	Estonia
1950	...	174.3	172.6	181.9	180.8	162.4	170.8
1951	...	194.2	180.6	187.2	165.0	176.9	171.1
1952	...	180.7	168.4	190.7	170.9	153.2	184.7
1953	...	179.1	169.4	197.6	169.6	154.3	169.9
1954	...	181.4	165.2	201.7	169.2	150.2	169.2
1955	...	174.3	174.2	178.5	152.4	158.0	166.4
1956	...	176.2	172.2	179.3	152.5	156.6	149.2
1957	...	173.6	164.7	191.6	161.8	144.6	159.4
1958	...	168.2	162.8	175.6	159.1	151.0	156.6
1959	...	166.3	155.0	184.2	160.1	148.0	157.7
1960	...	168.3	169.4	170.2	163.1	144.8	153.5
1961	...	156.8	152.9	169.0	152.9	150.6	156.4
1962	...	168.9	161.8	190.8	156.7	149.0	166.3
1963	...	166.6	168.4	171.4	153.6	152.1	145.8
1964	...	157.1	149.7	166.0	154.8	134.1	140.0
1965	133.5	168.4	157.0	170.5	151.7	135.6	148.7
1966	137.5	158.5	158.4	166.8	156.6	138.3	148.8
1967	128.8	164.8	153.3	166.7	142.9	130.0	145.4
1968	140.4	163.9	166.4	174.8	136.7	139.8	144.8
1969	125.7	162.4	157.9	169.3	131.3	132.4	156.5
1970	133.1	162.2	152.6	176.9	128.7	131.8	152.4
1971	129.0	165.3	155.6	169.7	124.8	129.1	142.0
1972	124.4	155.0	149.1	165.5	125.6	133.2	143.3
1973	125.6	152.5	150.2	172.1	123.3	132.7	141.5
1974	130.1	153.2	148.2	173.9	122.6	130.1	138.0
1975	116.6	156.9	151.3	168.4	116.6	128.7	142.6
1976	121.9	158.6	148.0	168.4	123.0	133.6	151.1
1977	113.0	148.0	134.4	168.5	109.2	124.5	141.6
1978	109.5	153.4	139.7	164.6	112.8	123.5	148.1
1979	106.1	145.9	130.7	164.3	113.6	124.0	147.3
1980	105.9	146.0	132.0	175.0	114.6	119.2	142.4
1981	102.2	145.3	128.3	164.1	113.1	118.3	141.1
1982	107.4	140.5	127.0	163.3	108.5	117.3	143.1
1983	98.0	143.9	130.8	169.1	111.7	115.1	138.3
1984	97.2	133.3	123.3	164.5	108.1	109.5	146.5
1985	105.6	138.1	123.0	163.2	110.4	114.6	147.9
1986	96.0	132.1	122.6	163.6	105.8	110.4	136.3
1987	97.1	127.6	112.6	154.7	104.7	104.6	140.3
1988	95.7	123.9	108.4	149.4	104.2	104.8	144.1
1989	99.7	121.1	112.5	154.1	103.9	106.2	132.5
1990	91.9	119.5	106.5	149.2	106.1	103.7	136.6

ANNEX TABLE 2 (cont.)
FEMALE

Year	Finland	France	Germany East	Germany West	Hungary	Iceland	Ireland
1950	187.6	161.2	...	...	176.6	...	167.5
1951	196.7	177.8	...	...	193.4	...	197.4
1952	188.3	158.5	...	...	201.4	...	151.3
1953	199.7	175.0	...	...	224.0	...	158.0
1954	183.1	153.6	189.9	...	202.8	...	159.4
1955	198.0	157.3	176.5	...	176.9	...	172.3
1956	183.2	166.2	173.9	171.1	182.8	...	158.4
1957	186.3	155.0	178.3	178.4	195.7	...	158.0
1958	188.4	148.1	176.9	170.6	177.1	...	162.0
1959	176.1	146.6	184.4	166.1	187.3	...	158.3
1960	181.5	150.2	189.7	177.1	182.0	...	150.6
1961	186.6	137.9	178.2	165.1	168.9	138.7	164.6
1962	197.6	151.3	192.4	166.4	199.1	135.2	157.8
1963	183.9	152.9	172.8	171.8	168.0	128.8	162.4
1964	182.7	135.8	175.6	153.0	169.1	132.6	153.2
1965	198.3	141.8	179.1	161.1	184.3	130.4	151.9
1966	184.0	133.7	174.1	160.4	163.0	121.0	162.5
1967	178.2	135.8	170.6	156.5	171.7	132.2	140.4
1968	182.7	137.1	188.2	170.4	178.8	151.5	151.4
1969	183.2	134.8	183.5	162.6	168.4	145.5	151.4
1970	169.3	129.8	179.3	160.9	175.7	144.7	145.5
1971	171.3	132.1	178.8	159.4	169.8	127.9	139.9
1972	164.4	126.0	176.0	156.2	163.1	119.5	151.1
1973	152.8	129.3	172.2	154.3	165.1	111.5	146.1
1974	157.0	125.6	168.2	153.1	163.4	117.8	153.7
1975	144.4	125.9	180.6	153.8	167.9	98.8	142.1
1976	142.3	128.6	174.2	149.1	167.0	95.7	149.8
1977	133.5	116.0	164.6	139.4	159.9	104.8	143.6
1978	129.7	118.0	168.2	141.1	171.1	94.6	147.7
1979	126.6	114.7	166.2	136.2	158.0	90.4	141.8
1980	130.8	114.8	172.4	134.2	167.7	89.9	137.2
1981	128.3	116.6	167.9	134.2	161.4	106.2	133.1
1982	117.7	110.2	165.8	130.1	162.3	93.0	129.0
1983	120.2	114.3	159.7	129.3	166.0	93.7	134.0
1984	117.2	107.2	159.8	122.2	158.3	85.9	126.7
1985	126.4	108.5	166.1	123.4	161.3	95.3	130.5
1986	119.2	105.8	164.8	121.6	160.5	91.9	134.5
1987	118.8	98.3	156.4	115.4	153.3	90.1	121.7
1988	120.0	96.0	154.0	113.4	148.1	100.3	122.4
1989	120.4	95.9	148.2	114.3	150.5	96.5	126.4
1990	119.6	93.5	143.9	116.2	150.5	...	...

ANNEX TABLE 2 (cont.)
FEMALE

Year	Italy	Japan	Latvia	Luxem-burg	Nether-lands	New Zealand	Norway
1950	...	185.8	147.8	...	...	149.9	151.0
1951	...	177.3	147.9	...	...	153.1	138.7
1952	158.0	171.2	146.1	...	...	142.3	139.1
1953	152.4	187.3	152.2	197.8	...	132.1	140.1
1954	133.0	163.3	152.9	163.9	...	135.1	143.3
1955	148.7	160.7	143.3	162.6	...	132.4	141.9
1956	174.8	177.3	131.3	198.8	...	135.1	139.0
1957	156.0	187.7	137.0	171.8	...	142.2	143.1
1958	147.0	161.5	135.4	170.8	...	138.3	143.7
1959	142.4	164.5	152.4	170.6	...	138.9	140.5
1960	151.9	173.7	136.9	188.0	150.1	134.4	140.5
1961	144.6	173.7	141.7	168.0	144.1	136.9	144.1
1962	158.6	179.9	159.2	190.1	152.1	135.1	141.6
1963	159.7	163.6	141.9	172.3	148.2	134.3	157.5
1964	146.9	162.6	125.8	161.7	134.9	138.7	141.5
1965	158.8	173.6	136.3	175.3	138.7	134.6	136.7
1966	149.6	159.1	135.2	160.0	140.9	138.3	138.1
1967	156.1	157.8	139.3	170.6	131.3	127.3	131.1
1968	167.1	156.9	135.6	177.1	138.5	126.2	135.6
1969	156.8	151.5	140.5	168.0	137.0	130.9	131.6
1970	142.1	154.7	137.9	157.9	135.0	131.3	133.1
1971	141.9	144.3	129.9	171.6	135.9	122.8	132.4
1972	136.8	139.6	134.0	145.5	136.6	131.1	131.7
1973	147.0	148.0	139.2	157.0	128.3	128.4	130.5
1974	139.0	146.4	133.6	153.3	123.7	124.2	126.3
1975	143.7	141.0	137.3	163.3	124.6	121.9	124.6
1976	140.5	139.4	138.1	166.2	121.8	118.7	123.3
1977	138.6	130.0	140.3	139.9	110.7	116.5	116.8
1978	132.7	126.6	142.1	146.5	114.2	108.3	116.4
1979	130.7	119.8	141.2	129.5	108.3	109.4	118.1
1980	133.0	124.1	140.8	150.6	106.8	118.1	112.7
1981	128.7	118.9	135.8	143.6	105.9	110.4	113.3
1982	122.2	111.0	129.7	134.0	105.4	108.2	105.7
1983	130.8	112.1	136.1	140.4	103.2	111.3	107.1
1984	118.1	106.7	140.8	129.3	102.6	102.6	106.2
1985	120.0	104.7	149.5	123.7	103.8	117.3	109.0
1986	117.1	100.1	136.5	129.1	105.2	109.7	103.3
1987	110.6	95.2	140.4	127.6	98.1	110.8	104.6
1988	111.0	98.1	138.1	105.0	100.0	111.7	107.3
1989	106.8	92.0	131.2	120.4	102.1	107.5	105.3
1990	...	92.5	142.4	...	...	101.1	...

ANNEX TABLE 2 (cont.)
FEMALE

Year	Poland	Portugal	Scotland	Singapore	Spain	Sweden	Switzerland
1950	...	150.8	181.4	...	150.7	177.0	169.8
1951	...	162.9	193.7	...	167.9	175.2	177.5
1952	...	154.1	172.0	...	140.0	164.3	164.0
1953	...	157.6	163.1	...	149.9	166.4	173.9
1954	...	156.8	172.8	...	142.1	166.7	166.9
1955	...	158.8	173.5	...	150.4	155.6	170.1
1956	...	191.7	175.6	...	165.3	157.4	173.3
1957	...	162.8	165.8	...	160.3	164.1	159.4
1958	...	147.4	169.3	...	144.7	157.1	155.5
1959	...	160.3	170.9	...	144.7	152.9	159.6
1960	...	163.1	164.9	...	146.9	158.2	165.0
1961	...	155.1	168.0	...	138.7	152.2	147.0
1962	...	151.9	158.5	...	148.8	157.6	163.8
1963	...	161.9	162.6	...	146.9	150.5	166.5
1964	...	155.0	144.2	...	139.7	143.5	146.6
1965	...	154.1	146.1	...	138.6	144.8	151.9
1966	...	161.2	153.7	...	137.7	141.5	152.5
1967	...	155.4	143.0	...	137.4	139.2	146.9
1968	...	152.6	150.9	...	139.0	143.6	152.5
1969	...	165.2	144.9	...	142.9	138.4	143.5
1970	...	151.2	143.4	...	137.9	127.4	143.0
1971	153.0	160.5	132.9	...	144.3	125.7	142.8
1972	142.4	147.0	142.1	...	134.7	124.5	133.9
1973	144.0	153.5	140.7	...	142.1	124.9	134.7
1974	141.2	159.1	141.1	...	138.7	121.0	129.4
1975	149.0	149.4	132.9	...	133.5	122.0	122.3
1976	144.8	156.4	139.3	...	132.4	125.6	125.5
1977	142.0	143.4	128.0	...	128.7	116.4	115.1
1978	146.3	149.2	132.2	...	126.4	115.9	118.5
1979	140.8	140.9	134.0	...	120.2	115.3	112.8
1980	152.6	139.1	124.2	...	118.6	115.4	115.2
1981	136.9	137.1	126.2	...	119.0	114.7	114.8
1982	136.3	129.9	130.8	117.5	111.2	108.5	112.3
1983	143.7	138.2	124.8	124.5	117.3	107.3	113.0
1984	150.7	137.4	118.8	115.6	111.4	104.6	104.3
1985	156.1	136.2	122.9	109.0	115.8	107.4	103.1
1986	150.3	131.3	121.8	101.3	111.7	105.5	104.0
1987	148.9	131.1	114.0	98.5	...	102.4	97.9
1988	140.7	132.1	114.1	105.7	...	106.3	97.4
1989	142.4	128.1	123.9	103.8	...	99.5	96.6
1990	141.7	139.8	114.3	101.0	...	102.0	99.4

ANNEX TABLE 3. AGE-STANDARDIZED DEATH RATES AT AGES 80-99 BY 5-YEAR PERIODS.

MALE

Year	Australia	Austria	Belgium	Czecho-slovakia	Denmark	England & Wales	Estonia
1950 - 1954	...	207.4	201.4	214.2	177.9	206.8	221.5
1955 - 1959	...	201.9	193.8	207.4	172.4	200.3	189.1
1960 - 1964	...	198.3	191.4	202.6	176.1	193.3	189.2
1965 - 1969	177.3	197.6	188.8	203.2	169.4	184.5	184.2
1970 - 1974	176.3	195.5	185.0	208.1	156.0	181.4	183.2
1975 - 1979	160.6	193.1	180.6	207.4	153.6	179.3	185.3
1980 - 1984	148.7	181.2	172.7	211.2	153.7	168.8	181.5
1985 - 1989	143.2	162.3	163.0	197.7	149.0	159.3	179.5

ANNEX TABLE 3 (cont.)

MALE

Year	Finland	France	Germany East	Germany West	Hungary	Iceland	Ireland
1950 - 1954	214.5	207.6	207.9	...	221.4	...	196.9
1955 - 1959	209.0	197.0	199.0	194.7	200.5	...	190.8
1960 - 1964	204.2	188.5	203.9	192.2	203.0	154.8	190.1
1965 - 1969	213.7	179.3	207.0	192.3	201.9	150.0	186.9
1970 - 1974	197.4	170.3	201.2	191.1	201.0	145.0	185.1
1975 - 1979	178.0	166.7	204.0	184.6	201.3	121.9	186.8
1980 - 1984	165.0	158.2	205.1	173.0	204.9	127.3	181.3
1985 - 1989	161.9	145.9	199.7	161.8	195.8	125.4	174.5

ANNEX TABLE 3 (cont.)

MALE

Year	Italy	Japan	Latvia	Luxem-burg	Nether-lands	New Zealand	Norway
1950 - 1954	166.9	214.1	187.2	211.0	...	167.9	155.3
1955 - 1959	176.7	209.6	172.3	209.1	...	168.4	153.4
1960 - 1964	177.9	213.0	167.1	203.6	163.8	173.4	163.2
1965 - 1969	187.3	200.8	165.0	194.8	158.0	173.4	159.4
1970 - 1974	172.1	184.5	165.2	198.1	156.8	172.0	158.8
1975 - 1979	174.3	166.0	174.0	193.0	152.4	165.4	152.3
1980 - 1984	165.4	150.8	168.2	181.3	148.8	159.8	148.0
1985 - 1989	152.2	137.6	174.7	175.7	150.7	155.8	147.8

ANNEX TABLE 3 (cont.)

MALE

Year	Poland	Portugal	Scotland	Singa-pore	Spain	Sweden	Switzer-land
1950 - 1954	...	198.8	218.9	...	186.9	182.8	197.2
1955 - 1959	...	207.5	210.1	...	187.9	174.9	190.6
1960 - 1964	...	199.9	205.6	...	179.5	174.1	185.6
1965 - 1969	...	201.4	194.3	...	173.0	167.9	179.8
1970 - 1974	178.7	194.1	192.3	...	172.7	159.4	168.6
1975 - 1979	179.8	186.7	189.7	...	159.5	160.6	158.5
1980 - 1984	180.1	174.6	182.4	153.3	143.6	154.0	153.1
1985 - 1989	186.0	170.5	174.6	132.0	140.7	149.5	142.3

ANNEX TABLE 3 (cont.)

FEMALE

Year	Australia	Austria	Belgium	Czecho-slovakia	Denmark	England & Wales	Estonia
1950 - 1954	...	182.0	171.3	191.8	171.1	159.4	173.1
1955 - 1959	...	171.7	165.8	181.8	157.2	151.6	157.9
1960 - 1964	...	163.5	160.4	173.5	156.2	146.1	152.4
1965 - 1969	133.2	163.6	158.6	169.6	143.8	135.2	148.8
1970 - 1974	128.4	157.7	151.1	171.6	125.0	131.4	143.4
1975 - 1979	113.4	152.6	140.8	166.8	115.0	126.9	146.2
1980 - 1984	102.1	141.8	128.3	167.2	111.2	115.9	142.3
1985 - 1989	98.8	128.5	115.8	157.0	105.8	108.1	140.2

ANNEX TABLE 3 (cont.)

FEMALE

Year	Finland	France	Germany East	Germany West	Hungary	Iceland	Ireland
1950 - 1954	191.1	165.2	189.9	...	199.6	...	166.7
1955 - 1959	186.4	154.6	178.0	171.6	184.0	...	161.8
1960 - 1964	186.4	145.6	181.7	166.7	177.4	133.8	157.7
1965 - 1969	185.3	136.7	179.1	162.2	173.2	136.1	151.5
1970 - 1974	163.0	128.6	174.9	156.8	167.4	124.3	147.3
1975 - 1979	135.3	120.6	170.8	143.9	164.8	96.9	145.0
1980 - 1984	122.8	112.6	165.1	130.0	163.1	93.7	132.0
1985 - 1989	121.0	100.9	157.9	117.6	154.7	94.8	127.1

ANNEX TABLE 3 (cont.)

FEMALE

Year	Italy	Japan	Latvia	Luxem-burg	Nether-lands	New Zealand	Norway
1950 - 1954	147.8	177.0	149.4	180.9	...	142.5	142.4
1955 - 1959	153.8	170.3	139.9	174.9	...	137.4	141.6
1960 - 1964	152.3	170.7	141.1	176.0	145.9	135.9	145.0
1965 - 1969	157.7	159.8	137.4	170.2	137.3	131.4	134.6
1970 - 1974	141.4	146.6	134.9	157.1	131.9	127.6	130.8
1975 - 1979	137.2	131.4	139.8	149.1	115.9	115.0	119.9
1980 - 1984	126.5	114.6	136.6	139.6	104.8	110.1	109.0
1985 - 1989	113.1	98.0	139.1	121.1	101.9	111.4	105.9

ANNEX TABLE 3 (cont.)

FEMALE

Year	Poland	Portugal	Scotland	Singa-pore	Spain	Sweden	Switzer-land
1950 - 1954	...	156.4	176.6	...	150.1	169.9	170.4
1955 - 1959	...	164.2	171.0	...	153.1	157.4	163.6
1960 - 1964	...	157.4	159.6	...	144.2	152.4	157.8
1965 - 1969	...	157.7	147.7	...	139.1	141.5	149.5
1970 - 1974	145.2	154.3	140.0	...	139.5	124.7	136.8
1975 - 1979	144.6	147.8	133.3	...	128.2	119.0	118.8
1980 - 1984	144.0	136.3	125.0	119.1	115.5	110.1	111.9
1985 - 1989	147.7	131.7	119.4	103.7	113.7	104.2	99.8

ANNEX TABLE 4. AGE-STANDARDIZED DEATH RATES AT AGES 80-99
IN SELECTED GROUPS OF COUNTRIES.

MALES

Year	High mortality (3 countries)	Medium mortality (5 countries)	Low mortality (4 countries)	Rapid decline (2 countries)	Western Europe (11 countries)
1950	...	...	184.5	202.2	...
1951	...	...	175.8	219.1	...
1952	...	...	172.9	199.6	...
1953	...	...	172.7	215.3	...
1954	213.2	...	170.0	197.2	...
1955	195.6	...	165.7	200.7	...
1956	200.3	201.8	169.1	210.4	199.9
1957	207.5	196.0	173.0	198.2	193.6
1958	197.6	196.1	171.0	187.4	190.3
1959	206.8	192.0	167.8	185.7	187.0
1960	207.8	196.1	171.6	192.4	191.9
1961	197.0	190.4	165.9	178.6	183.9
1962	221.9	196.6	174.2	196.4	193.6
1963	194.4	203.0	175.0	196.7	197.5
1964	195.8	179.9	162.3	177.0	176.8
1965	208.2	188.2	166.8	185.3	184.6
1966	195.1	189.3	166.9	172.8	181.7
1967	198.7	183.2	158.7	177.6	178.4
1968	213.8	197.7	165.4	181.1	188.8
1969	208.9	189.0	162.2	179.7	182.8
1970	204.9	186.4	157.7	171.4	178.4
1971	203.9	186.8	159.9	174.0	179.7
1972	199.6	187.8	159.4	166.3	178.0
1973	205.2	187.9	159.4	172.0	179.7
1974	201.4	185.7	156.4	167.0	176.6
1975	209.0	189.2	159.7	169.4	179.8
1976	205.8	188.7	161.7	178.3	182.2
1977	199.4	177.0	150.5	159.0	168.5
1978	203.7	180.1	154.3	164.2	172.3
1979	203.8	177.1	153.3	159.1	168.9
1980	213.8	174.8	153.5	160.1	167.9
1981	206.0	174.7	154.7	162.3	168.6
1982	205.6	171.7	150.5	155.0	164.2
1983	205.1	172.3	151.4	159.7	166.0
1984	202.7	164.2	149.3	151.7	158.7
1985	207.5	169.4	153.5	155.9	163.5
1986	205.3	164.7	150.3	150.6	158.9
1987	194.1	157.0	148.7	143.5	152.1
1988	192.9	155.3	150.6	139.8	150.3
1989	191.8	157.8	148.7	138.4	151.2
1990	190.4	155.9	...	137.4	...

ANNEX TABLE 4 (Cont.).

FEMALES

Year	High mortality (3 countries)	Medium mortality (5 countries)	Low mortality (4 countries)	Rapid decline (2 countries)	Western Europe (11 countries)
1950	...	...	172.1	161.9	...
1951	...	...	164.1	177.7	...
1952	...	...	160.3	159.0	...
1953	...	...	161.3	174.9	...
1954	195.8	...	162.0	154.7	...
1955	177.1	...	151.6	158.4	...
1956	177.2	165.6	151.9	166.8	164.1
1957	185.5	162.9	158.6	155.3	160.2
1958	176.6	161.9	154.6	148.7	157.3
1959	185.0	157.8	152.0	147.7	154.2
1960	182.9	162.5	154.1	151.4	158.3
1961	173.8	158.0	148.8	138.6	151.3
1962	193.4	159.4	153.8	152.4	156.7
1963	171.4	163.1	151.9	154.1	159.1
1964	171.7	145.6	142.6	136.7	142.7
1965	177.9	151.2	143.2	142.7	147.7
1966	169.8	151.3	144.0	135.3	145.8
1967	169.8	146.0	136.3	136.7	142.1
1968	182.6	157.0	140.0	138.4	149.6
1969	176.5	149.9	136.4	135.6	144.1
1970	177.9	148.2	132.0	130.9	141.2
1971	174.4	146.9	131.0	133.0	140.9
1972	170.5	146.0	131.0	126.7	138.6
1973	170.7	144.8	127.4	129.8	138.3
1974	168.7	143.1	123.7	125.9	135.7
1975	174.7	143.1	123.1	125.6	135.5
1976	171.2	142.9	124.0	128.3	136.3
1977	164.7	133.1	113.6	116.0	125.8
1978	167.8	134.1	115.4	118.0	127.1
1979	163.9	131.0	113.4	114.5	124.1
1980	172.1	128.3	112.2	114.8	122.4
1981	165.5	127.6	111.5	116.5	122.4
1982	164.4	124.8	107.4	110.4	118.5
1983	163.6	124.1	107.0	114.2	119.1
1984	160.7	117.5	105.2	106.9	112.9
1985	164.3	120.6	107.3	108.1	115.3
1986	163.6	117.5	105.6	105.6	112.6
1987	155.3	111.4	102.0	98.2	106.5
1988	151.5	110.1	104.2	96.1	105.4
1989	150.3	111.2	102.6	96.0	105.8
1990	146.7	110.5	...	94.0	...

ANNEX TABLE 5. AGE-STANDARDIZED DEATH RATES AT AGES 80-99. AVERAGE OF LAST FIVE ANNUAL RATES.
MALE

Year	Australia	Austria	Belgium	Czecho-slovakia	Denmark	England & Wales	Estonia
1954	...	207.4	201.4	214.2	177.9	206.8	221.5
1955	...	208.6	202.7	212.9	173.7	207.0	216.1
1956	...	207.8	201.1	211.4	173.6	203.4	208.1
1957	...	206.2	199.5	212.5	173.7	201.4	197.1
1958	...	204.3	196.2	208.8	173.6	201.7	191.1
1959	...	201.9	193.8	207.4	172.4	200.3	189.1
1960	...	201.4	192.0	208.0	174.1	196.4	186.0
1961	...	197.4	188.9	206.1	174.7	194.2	191.5
1962	...	198.4	189.3	207.4	175.4	195.5	195.1
1963	...	199.9	192.4	206.1	175.2	196.3	195.7
1964	...	198.3	191.4	202.6	176.1	193.3	189.2
1965	...	197.5	188.7	202.6	175.7	192.3	191.3
1966	...	197.8	188.9	203.7	177.8	191.1	188.1
1967	...	196.8	187.2	199.0	175.0	186.7	183.2
1968	...	195.9	186.4	201.2	172.4	184.2	180.5
1969	177.3	197.6	188.8	203.2	169.3	184.5	184.2
1970	178.8	197.6	188.5	204.8	165.1	183.6	181.7
1971	177.6	199.7	188.9	206.5	160.5	181.3	180.5
1972	178.0	198.4	188.5	206.5	158.0	183.0	181.9
1973	173.9	196.4	186.5	206.8	156.4	181.2	183.5
1974	176.3	195.5	185.0	208.1	156.0	181.5	183.2
1975	173.1	195.5	186.9	208.4	155.7	181.9	183.1
1976	172.6	194.5	187.4	208.2	156.3	183.7	185.4
1977	169.7	193.2	185.2	210.0	154.8	181.6	181.2
1978	167.1	194.4	182.6	208.7	153.8	180.2	182.2
1979	160.6	193.1	180.6	207.4	153.7	179.3	185.3
1980	157.8	190.0	177.2	209.3	154.3	177.5	187.0
1981	153.3	188.6	173.8	209.2	153.3	174.2	186.1
1982	152.8	187.2	173.3	209.3	154.4	173.5	188.0
1983	150.4	184.3	173.8	211.1	155.1	172.1	184.5
1984	148.7	181.3	172.7	211.2	153.7	168.8	181.5
1985	149.1	179.3	171.6	207.9	153.2	168.2	181.3
1986	146.8	175.1	171.5	207.7	151.2	166.6	179.7
1987	143.7	170.8	168.9	204.1	150.7	163.3	180.7
1988	142.5	165.5	164.2	199.6	150.0	160.3	181.5
1989	143.2	162.3	163.0	197.7	148.9	159.3	179.5
1990	139.1	156.7	160.4	195.5	148.7	156.0	177.7

ANNEX TABLE 5 (cont.).

MALE

Year	Finland	France	Germany East	Germany West	Hungary	Iceland	Ireland
1954	214.5	207.6	...	...	221.4	...	196.9
1955	216.3	207.1	...	...	222.6	...	196.7
1956	215.1	205.2	...	...	218.4	...	187.6
1957	215.1	205.0	...	...	214.4	...	188.2
1958	211.5	199.3	199.8	...	202.8	...	190.7
1959	208.9	197.0	199.0	...	200.5	...	190.8
1960	204.9	195.4	202.4	196.1	203.1	...	186.1
1961	202.3	189.0	203.0	194.1	200.8	...	189.7
1962	202.6	188.7	206.0	192.8	205.4	...	192.2
1963	203.0	190.3	205.2	194.6	205.9	...	191.8
1964	204.2	188.5	203.9	192.2	203.0	...	190.1
1965	207.9	186.9	203.6	189.9	204.1	152.3	190.7
1966	210.9	185.5	202.9	190.4	202.8	153.7	191.7
1967	209.2	181.8	199.3	188.9	195.6	155.8	186.6
1968	211.4	178.7	203.9	189.1	199.7	152.7	185.8
1969	213.7	179.3	207.0	192.3	201.9	150.0	187.0
1970	210.9	176.5	205.5	192.5	200.5	149.7	186.7
1971	209.5	176.9	206.8	193.3	203.6	150.1	180.0
1972	206.9	174.5	206.9	194.2	204.1	149.4	183.3
1973	201.3	172.8	204.1	192.2	202.6	149.0	183.9
1974	197.3	170.3	201.2	191.1	201.0	145.0	185.1
1975	193.6	170.1	202.9	191.8	200.3	142.8	183.9
1976	189.9	171.2	203.5	191.1	200.8	134.2	188.0
1977	186.3	169.9	202.5	188.8	200.7	128.8	188.6
1978	183.7	168.3	202.4	187.0	201.3	122.0	187.9
1979	178.0	166.7	204.0	184.6	201.3	121.9	186.8
1980	176.4	164.7	204.3	180.7	202.9	122.4	188.6
1981	172.6	161.4	204.6	178.4	202.3	127.2	186.9
1982	168.2	160.5	206.4	177.0	203.7	127.5	184.8
1983	166.8	159.6	206.2	175.1	203.4	131.9	183.7
1984	165.0	158.2	205.1	173.0	204.9	127.3	181.3
1985	164.8	157.5	204.6	171.4	204.1	125.9	180.5
1986	163.1	155.2	204.5	169.0	204.0	121.8	181.3
1987	163.7	152.9	202.9	166.5	201.7	122.8	178.9
1988	162.0	148.8	201.9	163.1	198.1	121.2	176.1
1989	161.8	146.0	199.7	161.8	195.8	125.4	174.5
1990	158.9	141.9	195.6	160.1	192.6	...	...

ANNEX TABLE 5 (cont.).

MALE

Year	Italy	Japan	Latvia	Luxem-burg	Nether-lands	New Zealand	Norway
1954	...	214.1	187.2	...	...	167.9	155.3
1955	...	208.2	185.3	...	...	164.3	151.7
1956	174.1	209.5	181.5	...	...	164.5	152.6
1957	174.7	215.2	179.9	212.4	...	165.8	152.6
1958	173.9	209.0	174.0	207.3	...	166.5	152.8
1959	176.7	209.6	172.3	209.1	...	168.4	153.4
1960	178.3	213.8	169.1	214.1	...	170.6	155.5
1961	172.0	213.6	168.0	209.5	...	168.5	157.1
1962	173.0	212.7	168.8	213.3	...	169.4	159.0
1963	176.4	213.2	171.0	210.1	...	172.3	162.3
1964	177.9	212.9	167.1	203.6	163.8	173.4	163.2
1965	179.4	213.0	167.5	202.4	162.7	173.9	162.7
1966	181.5	209.1	166.5	201.4	162.7	176.6	162.8
1967	181.2	203.0	164.0	193.0	158.3	172.7	161.6
1968	183.7	202.6	163.3	190.2	156.6	174.3	159.0
1969	187.3	200.7	165.0	194.8	158.0	173.4	159.4
1970	184.3	196.0	166.4	192.0	157.4	174.2	160.0
1971	182.8	193.3	166.1	193.5	157.2	173.3	159.4
1972	179.3	189.6	165.6	192.2	159.6	175.3	160.0
1973	175.6	186.8	166.6	196.5	158.3	172.8	160.2
1974	172.1	184.5	165.2	198.1	156.8	172.0	158.8
1975	173.7	181.1	166.0	193.8	157.2	171.5	157.9
1976	174.9	179.6	168.8	197.6	157.4	171.3	157.0
1977	176.8	176.6	170.4	197.8	154.0	171.7	155.0
1978	175.0	171.8	170.6	197.5	153.2	168.1	153.2
1979	174.3	166.0	174.0	193.0	152.4	165.4	152.3
1980	173.3	162.8	173.2	193.7	149.9	166.8	150.7
1981	171.5	158.7	172.3	188.0	148.1	163.4	150.5
1982	168.3	155.0	170.1	184.1	148.9	160.7	149.8
1983	168.0	152.5	169.0	182.0	148.3	161.1	148.7
1984	165.4	150.7	168.2	181.3	148.8	159.8	148.0
1985	162.5	147.3	170.7	180.4	149.7	156.9	148.4
1986	160.1	143.9	170.9	179.6	150.2	157.1	146.6
1987	157.9	141.6	173.2	180.0	149.7	156.6	147.4
1988	154.2	139.6	175.5	176.2	149.6	156.3	147.7
1989	152.2	137.6	174.7	175.7	150.7	155.8	147.9
1990	...	136.0	174.3	...	...	151.3	...

ANNEX TABLE 5 (cont.).

MALE

Year	Poland	Portugal	Scotland	Singa-pore	Spain	Sweden	Switzer-land
1954	...	198.8	219.0	...	186.9	182.8	197.2
1955	...	200.5	217.3	...	186.0	179.2	199.4
1956	...	207.5	212.9	...	185.3	176.2	198.3
1957	...	210.7	210.2	...	190.0	176.2	198.1
1958	...	207.3	212.0	...	187.8	175.4	193.4
1959	...	207.5	210.1	...	187.9	174.9	190.6
1960	...	208.3	207.2	...	188.0	176.1	188.3
1961	...	198.6	207.3	...	180.6	175.0	182.4
1962	...	196.4	207.3	...	178.0	174.3	182.1
1963	...	201.8	208.9	...	179.6	174.8	185.8
1964	...	199.9	205.6	...	179.5	174.1	185.6
1965	...	198.6	205.5	...	177.3	172.9	185.4
1966	...	201.2	203.7	...	177.7	172.2	187.0
1967	...	201.3	199.0	...	174.8	169.7	183.0
1968	...	197.7	193.5	...	173.1	168.2	180.1
1969	...	201.4	194.3	...	173.0	167.9	179.8
1970	...	199.7	192.8	...	172.3	164.7	177.2
1971	...	198.4	188.4	...	174.7	163.3	175.9
1972	...	196.2	191.9	...	174.0	161.9	175.0
1973	...	196.4	192.6	...	174.2	160.5	171.2
1974	...	194.1	192.3	...	172.7	159.4	168.6
1975	178.8	193.8	192.1	...	172.7	160.7	166.2
1976	176.4	193.2	195.0	...	168.8	161.9	164.3
1977	177.3	193.8	191.5	...	167.4	162.1	161.6
1978	178.8	191.7	190.5	...	163.7	161.1	160.4
1979	179.8	186.8	189.7	...	159.5	160.6	158.5
1980	182.0	184.9	188.8	...	155.5	160.0	157.8
1981	180.8	180.7	186.5	...	152.0	158.4	156.1
1982	179.7	176.3	187.2	...	147.8	157.1	155.6
1983	178.4	174.3	185.8	...	145.6	156.2	155.1
1984	180.1	174.6	182.4	...	143.6	154.0	153.1
1985	181.3	174.2	180.3	...	142.8	153.0	151.1
1986	184.1	172.7	179.2	146.4	141.0	151.5	148.4
1987	186.9	172.3	176.0	141.8	...	150.8	145.9
1988	187.1	172.3	173.3	136.9	...	150.6	143.1
1989	186.0	170.5	174.6	132.1	...	149.5	142.3
1990	183.0	171.4	172.2	128.3	...	147.5	142.1

ANNEX TABLE 5 (cont.).

FEMALE

Year	Australia	Austria	Belgium	Czecho-slovakia	Denmark	England & Wales	Estonia
1954	...	181.9	171.2	191.8	171.1	159.4	173.1
1955	...	181.9	171.6	191.1	165.4	158.5	172.3
1956	...	178.3	169.9	189.6	162.9	154.5	167.9
1957	...	176.9	169.1	189.7	161.1	152.7	162.8
1958	...	174.7	167.8	185.3	159.0	152.1	160.2
1959	...	171.7	165.8	181.8	157.2	151.6	157.9
1960	...	170.5	164.8	180.2	159.3	149.0	155.3
1961	...	166.6	161.0	178.1	159.4	147.8	156.7
1962	...	165.7	160.4	178.0	158.4	148.7	158.1
1963	...	165.4	161.5	177.1	157.3	148.9	155.9
1964	...	163.5	160.4	173.5	156.2	146.1	152.4
1965	...	163.6	158.0	173.5	153.9	144.3	151.4
1966	...	163.9	159.1	173.1	154.7	141.8	149.9
1967	...	163.1	157.4	168.3	151.9	138.0	145.7
1968	...	162.5	157.0	169.0	148.5	135.6	145.5
1969	133.2	163.6	158.6	169.6	143.8	135.2	148.8
1970	133.1	162.4	157.7	170.9	139.2	134.5	149.6
1971	131.4	163.7	157.2	171.5	132.9	132.6	148.2
1972	130.5	161.8	156.3	171.2	129.4	133.3	147.8
1973	127.6	159.5	153.1	170.7	126.7	131.8	147.1
1974	128.4	157.6	151.1	171.6	125.0	131.4	143.4
1975	125.1	156.6	150.9	169.9	122.6	130.8	141.5
1976	123.7	155.2	149.4	169.7	122.2	131.7	143.3
1977	121.4	153.8	146.4	170.3	118.9	129.9	143.0
1978	118.2	154.0	144.3	168.8	116.8	128.1	144.3
1979	113.4	152.6	140.8	166.8	115.0	126.9	146.1
1980	111.3	150.4	137.0	168.2	114.6	125.0	146.1
1981	107.3	147.7	133.0	167.3	112.7	121.9	144.1
1982	106.2	146.2	131.5	166.3	112.5	120.5	144.4
1983	103.9	144.3	129.8	167.2	112.3	118.8	142.4
1984	102.1	141.8	128.3	167.2	111.2	115.9	142.3
1985	102.1	140.2	126.5	164.8	110.4	115.0	143.4
1986	100.8	137.6	125.3	164.7	108.9	113.4	142.4
1987	98.8	135.0	122.5	163.0	108.1	110.8	141.9
1988	98.3	131.0	118.0	159.1	106.6	108.8	143.0
1989	98.8	128.6	115.8	157.0	105.8	108.1	140.2
1990	96.1	124.8	112.5	154.2	104.9	105.9	138.0

ANNEX TABLE 5 (cont.).

FEMALE

Year	Finland	France	Germany East	Germany West	Hungary	Iceland	Ireland
1954	191.1	165.2	...	...	199.6	...	166.7
1955	193.2	164.4	...	...	199.7	...	167.7
1956	190.5	162.1	...	...	197.6	...	159.9
1957	190.1	161.4	...	...	196.4	...	161.2
1958	187.8	156.0	179.1	...	187.1	...	162.0
1959	186.4	154.6	178.0	...	184.0	...	161.8
1960	183.1	153.2	180.6	172.7	185.0	...	157.5
1961	183.8	147.6	181.5	171.5	182.2	...	158.7
1962	186.0	146.8	184.3	169.1	182.9	...	158.7
1963	185.1	147.8	183.5	169.3	181.1	...	158.7
1964	186.5	145.6	181.7	166.7	177.4	...	157.7
1965	189.8	143.9	179.6	163.5	177.9	133.1	158.0
1966	189.3	143.1	178.8	162.5	176.7	129.6	157.6
1967	185.4	140.0	174.4	160.6	171.2	129.0	154.1
1968	185.2	136.8	177.5	160.3	173.4	133.5	151.9
1969	185.3	136.6	179.1	162.2	173.2	136.1	151.5
1970	179.5	134.2	179.1	162.2	171.5	139.0	150.2
1971	176.9	133.9	180.1	162.0	172.9	140.4	145.7
1972	174.2	132.0	181.2	161.9	171.2	137.8	147.9
1973	168.2	130.4	178.0	158.7	168.4	129.8	146.8
1974	163.0	128.6	174.9	156.8	167.4	124.3	147.3
1975	158.0	127.8	175.2	155.4	165.9	115.1	146.6
1976	152.2	127.1	174.2	153.3	165.3	108.7	148.6
1977	146.0	125.1	172.0	149.9	164.7	105.7	147.1
1978	141.4	122.8	171.2	147.3	165.9	102.3	147.4
1979	135.3	120.6	170.8	143.9	164.8	96.9	145.0
1980	132.6	118.4	169.1	140.0	164.7	95.1	144.0
1981	129.8	116.0	167.9	137.0	163.6	97.2	140.7
1982	126.6	114.9	168.1	135.2	164.1	94.8	137.8
1983	124.7	114.1	166.4	132.8	163.1	94.6	135.0
1984	122.8	112.6	165.1	130.0	163.1	93.7	132.0
1985	122.0	111.4	163.9	127.8	161.9	94.8	130.7
1986	120.1	109.2	163.2	125.3	161.7	92.0	130.9
1987	120.4	106.8	161.4	122.4	159.9	91.4	129.5
1988	120.3	103.2	160.2	119.2	156.3	92.7	127.2
1989	121.0	100.9	157.9	117.6	154.7	94.8	127.1
1990	119.6	97.9	153.5	116.2	152.6	...	...

ANNEX TABLE 5 (cont.).

FEMALE

Year	Italy	Japan	Latvia	Luxem-burg	Nether-lands	New Zealand	Norway
1954	...	177.0	149.4	...	...	142.5	142.4
1955	...	172.0	148.5	...	...	139.0	140.6
1956	153.4	172.0	145.2	...	...	135.4	140.7
1957	153.0	175.3	143.3	179.0	...	135.4	141.5
1958	151.9	170.1	140.0	173.6	...	136.6	142.2
1959	153.8	170.3	139.9	174.9	...	137.4	141.6
1960	154.4	172.9	138.6	180.0	...	137.8	141.4
1961	148.4	172.2	140.7	173.8	...	138.1	142.4
1962	148.9	170.7	145.1	177.5	...	136.7	142.1
1963	151.4	171.1	146.4	177.8	...	135.9	144.8
1964	152.3	170.7	141.1	176.0	145.9	135.9	145.0
1965	153.7	170.7	141.0	173.5	143.6	135.9	144.3
1966	154.7	167.8	139.7	171.9	143.0	136.2	143.1
1967	154.2	163.3	135.7	168.0	138.8	134.6	141.0
1968	155.7	162.0	134.4	168.9	136.9	133.0	136.6
1969	157.7	159.8	137.4	170.2	137.3	131.5	134.6
1970	154.3	156.0	137.7	166.7	136.5	130.8	133.9
1971	152.8	153.0	136.6	169.0	135.5	127.7	132.8
1972	148.9	149.4	135.6	164.0	136.6	128.5	132.9
1973	144.9	147.6	136.3	160.0	134.6	128.9	131.9
1974	141.4	146.6	134.9	157.1	131.9	127.6	130.8
1975	141.7	143.9	134.8	158.1	129.8	125.7	129.1
1976	141.4	142.9	136.4	157.1	127.0	124.9	127.3
1977	141.8	141.0	137.7	155.9	121.8	121.9	124.3
1978	138.9	136.7	138.3	153.8	119.0	117.9	121.5
1979	137.2	131.4	139.8	149.1	115.9	115.0	119.8
1980	135.1	128.0	140.5	146.5	112.4	114.2	117.5
1981	132.7	123.9	140.0	142.0	109.2	112.5	115.5
1982	129.5	120.1	137.9	140.8	108.1	110.9	113.2
1983	129.1	117.2	136.7	139.6	105.9	111.5	111.4
1984	126.6	114.6	136.6	139.6	104.8	110.1	109.0
1985	124.0	110.7	138.4	134.2	104.2	110.0	108.3
1986	121.6	106.9	138.5	131.3	104.0	109.8	106.3
1987	119.3	103.8	140.7	130.0	102.6	110.3	106.0
1988	115.4	101.0	141.1	122.9	101.9	110.4	106.1
1989	113.1	98.0	139.1	121.2	101.8	111.4	105.9
1990	...	95.6	137.7	...	...	108.2	...

ANNEX TABLE 5 (cont.).

FEMALE

Year	Poland	Portugal	Scotland	Singa-pore	Spain	Sweden	Switzer-land
1954	...	156.4	176.6	...	150.1	169.9	170.4
1955	...	158.0	175.0	...	150.1	165.6	170.5
1956	...	163.8	171.4	...	149.5	162.1	169.6
1957	...	165.5	170.2	...	153.6	162.0	168.7
1958	...	163.5	171.4	...	152.6	160.2	165.0
1959	...	164.2	171.0	...	153.1	157.4	163.6
1960	...	165.1	169.3	...	152.4	157.9	162.6
1961	...	157.7	167.8	...	147.1	156.9	157.3
1962	...	155.6	166.3	...	144.8	155.6	158.2
1963	...	158.5	165.0	...	145.2	154.3	160.4
1964	...	157.4	159.6	...	144.2	152.4	157.8
1965	...	155.6	155.9	...	142.5	149.7	155.2
1966	...	156.8	153.0	...	142.3	147.6	156.3
1967	...	157.5	149.9	...	140.1	143.9	152.9
1968	...	155.7	147.6	...	138.5	142.5	150.1
1969	...	157.7	147.7	...	139.1	141.5	149.5
1970	...	157.1	147.2	...	139.0	138.0	147.7
1971	...	157.0	143.0	...	140.3	134.9	145.7
1972	...	155.3	142.8	...	139.8	131.9	143.1
1973	...	155.5	140.8	...	140.4	128.2	139.6
1974	...	154.3	140.0	...	139.5	124.7	136.8
1975	145.9	153.9	137.9	...	138.7	123.6	132.6
1976	144.3	153.1	139.2	...	136.3	123.6	129.2
1977	144.2	152.4	136.4	...	135.1	122.0	125.4
1978	144.7	151.5	134.7	...	131.9	120.2	122.2
1979	144.6	147.9	133.3	...	128.2	119.0	118.8
1980	145.3	145.8	131.5	...	125.3	117.7	117.4
1981	143.7	141.9	128.9	...	122.6	115.5	115.3
1982	142.6	139.2	129.5	...	119.1	114.0	114.7
1983	142.1	137.0	128.0	...	117.3	112.2	113.6
1984	144.0	136.3	125.0	...	115.5	110.1	111.9
1985	144.7	135.8	124.7	...	114.9	108.5	109.5
1986	147.4	134.6	123.8	113.6	113.5	106.7	107.3
1987	149.9	134.8	120.5	109.8	...	105.4	104.5
1988	149.3	133.6	118.3	106.0	...	105.2	101.3
1989	147.7	131.8	119.3	103.7	...	104.2	99.8
1990	144.8	132.5	117.6	102.1	...	103.1	99.1

ANNEX TABLE 6. MORTALITY OF THE ELDERLY IN 1955-59 AND 1985-89.
Central death rates per 1000 population. The rates for ages 60-79 are based on United Nations Demograp[hic] Yearbook, the other rates on the author's data.

Sex and age	France			Germany, West		
	1955-59	1985-89	Ratio	1955-59	1985-89	Ratio
Males						
60-64	25.88	18.60	0.629	25.42	19.40	0.763
65-69	38.18	29.55	0.774	39.16	30.35	0.775
70-74	59.56	39.45	0.662	61.82	50.87	0.823
75-79	95.54	68.40	0.716	100.30	82.80	0.826
80-84	154.8	111.7	0.722	153.6	128.2	0.835
85-89	239.8	177.8	0.741	241.5	194.0	0.803
90-94	352.1	275.5	0.782	350.6	288.4	0.823
95-99	450.9	390.1	0.865	461.3	385.6	0.836
100-	808.9	617.1	0.763	749.7	605.7	0.808
Females						
60-64	12.92	6.92	0.536	14.40	9.00	0.625
65-69	21.12	11.87	0.562	25.40	14.65	0.577
70-74	36.42	17.75	0.487	46.64	26.25	0.563
75-79	65.20	35.25	0.541	83.70	47.50	0.568
80-84	116.7	70.5	0.604	134.3	85.6	0.637
85-89	191.9	128.5	0.670	213.9	148.6	0.695
90-94	293.7	216.3	0.736	313.2	235.8	0.753
95-99	408.6	333.4	0.816	441.5	335.8	0.761
100-	695.6	479.8	0.690	681.2	486.5	0.714

Sex and age	Italy[1]			Japan		
	1955-59	1985-89	Ratio	1955-59	1985-89	Ratio
Males						
60-64	24.2	18.4	0.760	27.28	12.80	0.469
65-69	36.3	28.9	0.796	43.84	20.42	0.466
70-74	53.8	42.6	0.792	71.56	35.00	0.489
75-79	87.8	74.0	0.843	111.30	60.75	0.546
80-84	138.5	119.2	0.861	169.4	105.1	0.620
85-89	214.8	181.3	0.844	247.8	169.3	0.683
90-94	321.0	281.2	0.876	363.9	256.6	0.705
95-99	491.7	403.2	0.820	470.7	366.7	0.778
100-	561.3	584.6	0.977	550.3	497.9	0.905
Females						
60-64	12.6	7.7	0.610	16.98	6.12	0.360
65-69	21.8	13.2	0.606	28.48	10.20	0.358
70-74	38.9	21.9	0.563	49.44	18.45	0.373
75-79	70.1	42.6	0.607	81.16	34.97	0.431
80-84	115.9	81.3	0.701	132.5	68.6	0.518
85-89	187.2	141.4	0.755	206.6	124.2	0.601
90-94	281.9	235.2	0.834	308.3	210.7	0.683
95-99	441.2	357.3	0.810	450.1	327.4	0.727
100-	511.0	527.5	1.032	565.1	449.5	0.795

[1] For Italy, data for 1960-64 are substituted for 1955-59.

ANNEX TABLE 6 (cont.).

Sex and age	Denmark			Finland		
	1955-59	1985-89	Ratio	1955-59	1985-89	Ratio
Males						
60-64	19.14	21.30	1.113	32.74	23.70	0.724
65-69	30.68	32.70	1.066	48.62	36.00	0.740
70-74	49.02	50.27	1.025	73.12	56.10	0.767
75-79	79.94	78.50	0.982	111.26	85.90	0.772
80-84	132.2	118.6	0.897	167.6	128.5	0.767
85-89	210.9	175.8	0.834	250.6	194.9	0.778
90-94	321.6	265.0	0.824	360.5	279.4	0.775
95-99	451.0	391.1	0.867	463.0	411.0	0.888
Females						
60-64	13.12	11.93	0.909	15.44	8.67	0.562
65-69	22.46	17.13	0.763	28.38	15.40	0.543
70-74	39.76	27.27	0.686	49.92	27.53	0.551
75-79	71.60	44.23	0.618	89.96	50.03	0.556
80-84	119.2	75.9	0.637	145.3	89.0	0.613
85-89	193.8	132.3	0.683	226.9	150.1	0.662
90-94	297.5	220.7	0.742	340.4	241.4	0.709
95-99	423.8	335.3	0.791	440.0	365.1	0.830

Sex and age	Norway			Sweden		
Males						
60-64	17.64	17.90	1.015	18.24	13.32	0.730
65-69	27.12	28.90	1.066	29.42	25.35	0.861
70-74	44.10	46.47	1.054	48.32	42.20	0.873
75-79	71.68	72.66	1.014	80.28	67.77	0.844
80-84	114.3	116.2	1.017	133.1	114.6	0.861
85-89	189.2	177.8	0.990	216.5	181.9	0.840
90-94	301.9	262.3	0.869	325.2	282.1	0.867
95-99	443.1	396.1	0.893	467.0	398.8	0.854
Females						
60-64	10.60	8.23	0.776	12.38	7.90	0.638
65-69	18.86	12.80	0.679	21.84	12.57	0.576
70-74	33.84	22.93	0.678	39.34	22.00	0.559
75-79	61.10	42.00	0.687	69.34	39.20	0.565
80-84	105.8	75.4	0.713	119.8	73.0	0.609
85-89	174.2	134.2	0.770	192.8	133.0	0.690
90-94	280.2	220.3	0.786	297.9	221.2	0.743
95-99	399.0	334.8	0.839	432.2	342.7	0.793

ANNEX TABLE 6 (cont.).

Sex and age	Czechoslovakia[1]			Germany, East		
	1955-59	1985-89	Ratio	1955-59	1985-89	Ratio
Males						
60-64	27.06	31.20	1.153	23.58	23.00	0.97
65-69	41.94	45.30	1.080	36.78	36.60	0.99
70-74	64.98	69.02	1.062	57.88	62.95	1.08
75-79	98.78	105.67	1.070	95.10	101.35	1.06
80-84	158.7	160.9	1.014	155.3	157.9	1.01
85-89	245.0	231.7	0.946	242.2	240.8	0.99
90-94	359.6	329.9	0.917	359.5	352.9	0.98
95-99	541.2	509.8	0.942	483.4	479.2	0.99
Females						
60-64	13.80	13.25	0.961	13.86	11.90	0.85
65-69	24.32	22.20	0.913	24.04	20.10	0.83
70-74	43.58	40.47	0.929	43.80	37.95	0.86
75-79	76.72	69.20	0.902	80.62	66.65	0.82
80-84	133.6	119.3	0.893	137.5	117.6	0.85
85-89	212.7	193.1	0.908	218.2	197.9	0.90
90-94	318.0	294.1	0.925	320.1	302.5	0.94
95-99	449.1	442.0	0.984	479.8	438.2	0.91

Sex and age	Hungary			Netherlands[1]		
	1955-59	1985-89	Ratio	1955-59	1985-89	Ratio
Males						
60-64	25.10	33.02	1.316	20.04	18.05	0.90
65-69	39.32	44.76	1.138	31.32	30.12	0.96
70-74	61.40	67.56	1.100	46.94	48.87	1.04
75-79	99.10	100.56	1.015	76.78	78.60	1.02
80-84	157.5	157.8	1.002	126.3	120.1	0.95
85-89	243.8	231.6	0.950	198.6	180.5	0.90
90-94	356.4	340.8	0.956	304.1	263.6	0.86
95-99	479.5	447.0	0.932	448.2	356.4	0.79
Females						
60-64	16.40	14.60	0.890	10.60	8.10	0.76
65-69	28.70	23.18	0.808	18.90	12.92	0.68
70-74	49.64	40.18	0.809	34.74	22.12	0.63
75-79	86.26	67.02	0.777	62.88	39.62	0.63
80-84	144.1	118.3	0.821	110.7	72.7	0.65
85-89	220.9	189.7	0.859	179.4	128.0	0.71
90-94	335.1	287.8	0.859	274.5	214.2	0.78
95-99	470.4	420.7	0.894	408.6	320.4	0.78

[1] For Czechoslovakia and the Netherlands, data for 1960-64 are substituted for 1955-59.

ANNEX TABLE 7. DEATH RATES BY AGE AND SEX FOR GROUPS OF COUNTRIES.

HIGH MORTALITY GROUP

Sex and year	80-84	85-89	90-94	95-99	100 +
Male					
1950-1954	166.2	257.4	381.5	540.2	...
1955-1959	157.8	245.5	361.4	481.2	...
1960-1964	158.7	246.4	366.6	525.1	...
1965-1969	161.4	246.5	366.0	516.6	...
1970-1974	161.9	243.7	351.9	486.3	...
1975-1979	163.2	244.9	357.0	467.2	...
1980-1984	165.3	246.4	359.7	500.0	...
1985-1989	158.7	236.4	344.2	480.6	...
Female					
1950-1954	150.3	234.0	343.5	496.3	...
1955-1959	139.3	220.2	328.3	474.8	...
1960-1964	137.5	219.2	327.0	465.6	...
1965-1969	134.0	215.9	324.6	468.4	...
1970-1974	131.8	212.7	319.1	450.8	...
1975-1979	127.4	209.8	317.5	433.0	...
1980-1984	125.0	204.2	314.2	440.7	...
1985-1989	118.2	194.9	297.2	435.5	...

MEDIUM MORTALITY GROUP

Sex and year	80-84	85-89	90-94	95-99	100 +
Male					
1950-1954	160.9	249.5	350.3	...	...
1955-1959	155.9	242.4	349.8	476.9	668.1
1960-1964	152.9	233.7	336.5	473.7	657.3
1965-1969	151.3	227.3	328.4	447.3	603.6
1970-1974	149.8	222.7	323.9	446.2	652.7
1975-1979	146.0	216.9	317.3	448.7	626.4
1980-1984	137.5	204.1	296.8	416.1	591.5
1985-1989	128.2	192.6	280.7	389.4	555.8
Female					
1950-1954	133.8	211.2	297.8	...	...
1955-1959	126.1	202.4	297.2	424.4	567.3
1960-1964	120.8	194.5	291.0	410.1	531.7
1965-1969	115.2	186.3	281.4	400.4	526.7
1970-1974	110.2	180.2	275.8	401.2	588.6
1975-1979	102.3	169.6	264.6	388.6	564.7
1980-1984	92.5	154.8	243.4	355.5	517.6
1985-1989	83.8	143.1	227.3	329.1	478.4

ANNEX TABLE 7 (Cont.)

LOW MORTALITY GROUP

Sex and year	80-84	85-89	90-94	95-99	100 +
Male					
1950-1954	133.7	215.3	327.7	468.3	695.6
1955-1959	128.5	208.7	318.9	456.8	684.9
1960-1964	130.6	205.9	316.2	473.9	676.8
1965-1969	127.0	199.4	300.8	425.7	662.6
1970-1974	123.8	191.9	284.9	415.5	561.4
1975-1979	122.6	186.7	279.4	414.0	563.3
1980-1984	119.8	182.1	270.3	391.2	575.1
1985-1989	118.1	180.6	270.7	383.1	532.2
Female					
1950-1954	125.3	201.6	303.7	444.2	653.4
1955-1959	116.4	188.8	293.7	422.1	602.8
1960-1964	113.7	184.8	285.5	416.6	521.8
1965-1969	104.7	174.8	267.2	386.7	573.4
1970-1974	95.8	160.8	252.1	365.2	533.9
1975-1979	86.2	148.0	234.9	352.9	495.5
1980-1984	78.6	136.1	221.8	338.4	468.3
1985-1989	74.1	131.8	219.5	333.6	488.3

RAPID DECLINE GROUP

Sex and year	80-84	85-89	90-94	95-99	100 +
Male					
1950-1954	162.7	253.0	361.6	476.3	891.4
1955-1959	154.2	239.8	350.2	450.3	798.4
1960-1964	147.5	230.1	334.1	443.6	793.4
1965-1969	141.4	216.2	322.8	413.9	634.7
1970-1974	134.6	205.0	299.6	414.9	681.9
1975-1979	129.2	201.1	304.1	415.2	646.8
1980-1984	122.5	191.1	289.3	407.4	630.4
1985-1989	111.4	177.4	275.9	389.6	606.5
Female					
1950-1954	127.0	204.3	303.4	434.0	735.5
1955-1959	117.4	192.8	294.3	410.5	691.8
1960-1964	110.0	182.5	281.3	395.7	653.5
1965-1969	102.8	171.4	267.3	380.4	551.0
1970-1974	95.6	161.6	253.3	369.2	540.1
1975-1979	87.2	151.5	245.2	366.8	532.8
1980-1984	80.2	142.4	235.2	347.8	510.8
1985-1989	70.4	128.3	216.5	334.2	481.4

ANNEX TABLE 7 (Cont.)

WESTERN EUROPE

Sex and year	80-84	85-89	90-94	95-99	100 +
Male					
1950-1954	157.8	246.0	350.5	...	...
1955-1959	151.8	237.3	345.9	466.8	706.9
1960-1964	148.5	229.0	333.2	465.3	698.1
1965-1969	145.3	220.5	323.2	435.1	620.1
1970-1974	142.1	213.7	312.0	433.4	648.9
1975-1979	138.2	208.5	308.6	434.7	623.9
1980-1984	131.0	197.6	291.2	410.4	600.3
1985-1989	122.2	186.6	278.0	388.6	567.0
Female					
1950-1954	130.8	208.0	300.1	...	...
1955-1959	122.4	197.9	295.9	420.2	606.9
1960-1964	116.8	189.9	287.6	406.9	564.6
1965-1969	110.3	180.6	275.6	393.0	539.6
1970-1974	104.2	172.4	266.4	387.5	567.8
1975-1979	95.9	161.7	255.3	377.8	546.7
1980-1984	87.2	148.9	238.3	351.1	509.2
1985-1989	78.8	137.5	223.2	331.1	480.5

JAPAN

Sex and year	80-84	85-89	90-94	95-99	100 +
Male					
1950-1954	171.4	256.5	373.5	468.2	493.8
1955-1959	169.4	247.8	363.9	470.7	550.3
1960-1964	172.5	253.0	358.4	496.9	617.3
1965-1969	160.4	242.7	345.1	445.2	553.9
1970-1974	145.3	224.2	324.7	442.2	483.4
1975-1979	128.9	202.3	300.3	425.1	604.2
1980-1984	116.6	183.6	278.1	385.1	514.0
1985-1989	105.1	169.3	256.6	366.7	497.9
Female					
1950-1954	138.3	214.2	322.4	431.5	478.7
1955-1959	132.5	206.6	308.3	450.1	565.1
1960-1964	132.4	207.5	313.3	436.6	606.4
1965-1969	121.9	197.1	297.2	422.5	530.7
1970-1974	109.6	181.8	285.5	401.8	511.2
1975-1979	95.8	165.3	263.4	382.7	519.9
1980-1984	81.4	145.2	239.8	357.0	491.7
1985-1989	68.6	124.2	210.7	327.4	449.5

ANNEX TABLE 8. DEATHS PER 1000 POPULATION AGED 100 YEARS AND OVER, 1950-1989. Pooled data for 13 countries of Western Europe[1].

Year	Males			Females		
	Mean Population	Deaths	Rate per 1000	Mean Population	Deaths	Rate per 1000
1950	138	105	760.9	488	312	639.3
1951	141	106	751.8	518	329	635.1
1952	164	102	622.0	649	352	542.4
1953	171	132	771.9	673	453	673.1
1954	179	117	653.6	696	418	600.6
1955	173	132	763.0	769	440	572.2
1956	200	164	820.0	891	578	648.7
1957	214	142	663.6	970	563	580.4
1958	253	149	588.9	1062	593	558.4
1959	288	177	614.6	1165	682	585.4
1960	329	239	726.4	1314	727	553.3
1961	343	245	714.3	1489	803	539.3
1962	369	244	661.2	1631	977	599.0
1963	377	263	697.6	1702	1062	624.0
1964	436	267	612.4	1822	995	546.1
1965	468	301	643.2	1971	1068	541.9
1966	518	322	621.6	2161	1120	518.3
1967	561	350	623.9	2380	1190	500.0
1968	580	384	662.1	2483	1395	561.8
1969	626	389	621.4	2536	1431	564.3
1970	699	429	613.7	2755	1502	545.2
1971	740	480	648.6	2922	1599	547.2
1972	815	467	573.0	3298	1699	515.2
1973	881	583	661.7	3616	1897	524.6
1974	956	606	633.9	3926	2177	554.5
1975	1062	654	615.8	4187	2315	552.9
1976	1140	698	612.3	4494	2347	522.3
1977	1196	718	600.3	4879	2523	517.1
1978	1251	784	626.7	5225	2648	506.8
1979	1310	799	609.9	5547	2833	510.7
1980	1403	841	599.4	5930	3197	539.1
1981	1480	927	626.4	6455	3249	503.3
1982	1577	932	591.0	7188	3448	479.7
1983	1732	1014	585.5	7824	4017	513.4
1984	1851	1082	584.5	8458	4000	472.9
1985	1931	1079	558.8	9114	4611	505.9
1986	2029	1168	575.7	9802	4577	466.9
1987	2199	1168	531.2	10736	5036	469.1
1988	2393	1266	529.0	11803	5596	474.1
1989	2559	1317	514.7	12777	6137	480.3

[1] Austria, Belgium (1974-), Denmark, England & Wales, Finland, France, Germany West (1956-), Iceland, Italy (1952-), Netherlands (1960-), Norway, Sweden and Switzerland.

ANNEX TABLE 9. PROBABILITY OF DYING AT AGES 100 AND OVER.
Pooled data for 14 countries[1].

Age x	Males			Females		
	Reached age x	Died before age x+1	1000q	Reached age x	Died before age x+1	1000q
1950-1960						
100	1 642	820	499	5 894	2 593	440
101	770	336	426	3 045	1 334	438
102	401	189	471	1 561	694	445
103	191	94	492	782	383	490
104	94	46		362	173	478
105	45	24		160	80	500
106	21	12		69	32	
107	8	2		41	26	
108	6	5		12	7	
109	1	1		4	3	
1960-1970						
100	3 619	1 663	460	13 132	5 476	417
101	1 769	831	470	7 164	3 000	419
102	878	410	467	3 906	1 661	425
103	443	220	497	2 082	954	458
104	200	112	560	1 043	494	474
105	83	42		517	258	499
106	38	23		237	118	498
107	13	6		104	62	596
108	6	2		37	21	
109	4	2		15	12	
110	1	-		4	2	
111	1	1		1	1	

[1] The same 13 countries as in Annex Table 8 plus Japan.

ANNEX TABLE 9 (Cont.).

Age x	Males			Females		
	Reached age x	Died before age x+1	1000q	Reached age x	Died before age x+1	1000q
1970-1980						
100	7 611	3 449	453	27 514	10 881	395
101	3 915	1 796	459	15 413	6 305	409
102	1 992	911	457	8 428	3 581	425
103	1 004	494	492	4 437	1 939	437
104	478	235	492	2 298	1 077	469
105	233	126	541	1 116	558	500
106	100	49	490	509	260	511
107	45	23		239	126	527
108	18	11		109	67	614
109	7	6		36	24	
110	1	1		10	3	
111				7	4	
112				3	2	
113				1	1	
1980-1990						
100	13 433	5 658	421	56 926	20 927	368
101	7 293	3 097	425	33 003	12 646	383
102	3 856	1 657	430	18 547	7 363	397
103	2 032	942	464	10 249	4 308	420
104	1 007	445	442	5 382	2 332	433
105	495	223	451	2 759	1 267	459
106	243	110	453	1 342	610	455
107	109	53	486	644	307	477
108	53	29		297	167	562
109	19	15		116	70	603
110	5	2		40	21	
111	2	1		14	5	
112				6	2	
113				4	1	
114				3	1	

ANNEX TABLE 10. SEX RATIO OF MORTALITY AT AGES 80-99, BY COUNTRY.

Year	Australia	Austria	Belgium	Czecho-slovakia	Denmark	England & Wales	Estonia
1950-54	...	1.140	1.176	1.116	1.040	1.298	1.279
1955-59	...	1.176	1.169	1.141	1.097	1.321	1.198
1960-64	...	1.212	1.193	1.168	1.127	1.323	1.241
1965-69	1.332	1.208	1.190	1.198	1.178	1.364	1.238
1970-74	1.372	1.240	1.224	1.212	1.248	1.381	1.278
1975-79	1.416	1.266	1.283	1.243	1.335	1.413	1.268
1980-84	1.456	1.278	1.346	1.263	1.383	1.457	1.276
1985-89	1.450	1.263	1.407	1.259	1.408	1.473	1.280

Year	Finland	France	Germany East	Germany West	Hungary	Iceland	Ireland
1950-54	1.123	1.256	1.095	...	1.109	...	1.181
1955-59	1.121	1.274	1.118	1.135	1.090	...	1.179
1960-64	1.095	1.294	1.122	1.153	1.144	1.157	1.206
1965-69	1.153	1.312	1.156	1.186	1.166	1.102	1.234
1970-74	1.211	1.325	1.151	1.219	1.200	1.167	1.257
1975-79	1.316	1.382	1.195	1.283	1.221	1.259	1.288
1980-84	1.343	1.405	1.242	1.330	1.256	1.359	1.374
1985-89	1.338	1.446	1.265	1.376	1.265	1.323	1.373

ANNEX TABLE 10 (Cont.).

Year	Italy	Japan	Latvia	Luxemburg	Netherlands	New Zealand	Norway
1950-54	1.129	1.209	1.254	1.167	...	1.178	1.091
1955-59	1.149	1.231	1.232	1.195	...	1.226	1.083
1960-64	1.168	1.247	1.184	1.157	1.123	1.276	1.125
1965-69	1.188	1.256	1.201	1.145	1.151	1.319	1.184
1970-74	1.218	1.259	1.224	1.261	1.189	1.348	1.214
1975-79	1.270	1.263	1.244	1.295	1.314	1.439	1.271
1980-84	1.307	1.316	1.231	1.299	1.420	1.451	1.358
1985-89	1.346	1.404	1.256	1.450	1.480	1.398	1.396

Year	Poland	Portugal	Scotland	Singapore	Spain	Sweden	Switzerland
1950-54	...	1.271	1.240	...	1.245	1.076	1.157
1955-59	...	1.264	1.228	...	1.228	1.111	1.165
1960-64	...	1.270	1.288	...	1.245	1.142	1.176
1965-69	...	1.277	1.315	...	1.243	1.186	1.203
1970-74	1.231	1.258	1.374	...	1.237	1.278	1.233
1975-79	1.243	1.263	1.424	...	1.244	1.349	1.334
1980-84	1.251	1.281	1.459	1.275	1.243	1.399	1.368
1985-89	1.259	1.294	1.463	1.299	1.237	1.434	1.426

ANNEX TABLE 11. SEX RATIO OF MORTALITY BY AGE FOR GROUPS OF COUNTRIES.

HIGH MORTALITY GROUP

Year	80-84	85-89	90-94	95-99	100 +
1950-1954	1.106	1.100	1.111	1.088	...
1955-1959	1.133	1.115	1.101	1.013	...
1960-1964	1.154	1.124	1.121	1.128	...
1965-1969	1.204	1.142	1.128	1.103	...
1970-1974	1.228	1.146	1.103	1.079	...
1975-1979	1.281	1.167	1.124	1.079	...
1980-1984	1.322	1.207	1.145	1.135	...
1985-1989	1.343	1.213	1.158	1.104	...

MEDIUM MORTALITY GROUP

Year	80-84	85-89	90-94	95-99	100 +
1950-1954	1.203	1.181	1.176	1.208	1.204
1955-1959	1.236	1.198	1.177	1.124	1.178
1960-1964	1.266	1.202	1.156	1.155	1.236
1965-1969	1.313	1.220	1.167	1.117	1.146
1970-1974	1.359	1.236	1.174	1.112	1.109
1975-1979	1.427	1.279	1.199	1.155	1.109
1980-1984	1.486	1.318	1.219	1.170	1.143
1985-1989	1.530	1.346	1.235	1.183	1.162

LOW MORTALITY GROUP

Year	80-84	85-89	90-94	95-99	100 +
1950-1954	1.067	1.068	1.079	1.054	1.065
1955-1959	1.104	1.105	1.086	1.082	1.136
1960-1964	1.149	1.114	1.108	1.138	1.297
1965-1969	1.213	1.141	1.126	1.101	1.156
1970-1974	1.292	1.193	1.130	1.138	1.052
1975-1979	1.422	1.261	1.189	1.173	1.137
1980-1984	1.524	1.338	1.219	1.156	1.228
1985-1989	1.594	1.370	1.233	1.148	1.090

ANNEX TABLE 11 (Cont.).

RAPID DECLINE GROUP

Year	80-84	85-89	90-94	95-99	100 +
1950-1954	1.281	1.238	1.192	1.097	1.212
1955-1959	1.313	1.244	1.190	1.097	1.154
1960-1964	1.341	1.261	1.188	1.121	1.214
1965-1969	1.375	1.261	1.208	1.088	1.152
1970-1974	1.408	1.269	1.183	1.124	1.263
1975-1979	1.482	1.327	1.240	1.132	1.214
1980-1984	1.527	1.342	1.230	1.171	1.234
1985-1989	1.582	1.383	1.274	1.166	1.260

WESTERN EUROPE

Year	80-84	85-89	90-94	95-99	100 +
1950-1954	1.206	1.183	1.168	1.138	1.181
1955-1959	1.240	1.199	1.169	1.111	1.165
1960-1964	1.271	1.206	1.159	1.144	1.236
1965-1969	1.317	1.221	1.173	1.107	1.149
1970-1974	1.364	1.240	1.171	1.118	1.143
1975-1979	1.441	1.289	1.209	1.151	1.141
1980-1984	1.502	1.327	1.222	1.169	1.179
1985-1989	1.551	1.359	1.246	1.174	1.180

JAPAN

Year	80-84	85-89	90-94	95-99	100 +
1950-1954	1.239	1.197	1.158	1.085	1.032
1955-1959	1.278	1.199	1.180	1.046	0.974
1960-1964	1.303	1.219	1.144	1.138	1.018
1965-1969	1.316	1.231	1.161	1.054	1.044
1970-1974	1.326	1.233	1.137	1.101	0.946
1975-1979	1.346	1.224	1.140	1.111	1.162
1980-1984	1.432	1.264	1.160	1.079	1.045
1985-1989	1.532	1.363	1.218	1.120	1.108

ANNEX TABLE 12.   STANDARD POPULATION: SWEDEN, BOTH SEXES, 1950-1989

Age x	Reached age x 1950-88	Died before age x+1	Same divided by 2	Mean population	Weights
80	1316742	111318	55659	1261083	.1625
81	1172469	110039	55019	1117450	.1440
82	1030935	106380	53190	977745	.1260
83	897404	101452	50726	846678	.1091
84	776373	95985	47992	728380	.0938
85	656774	90418	45209	611565	.0788
86	549857	82348	41174	508683	.0655
87	451148	73699	36849	414298	.0534
88	364244	64990	32495	331749	.0428
89	287894	55309	27654	260240	.0335
90	224176	46564	23282	200894	.0259
91	170721	38359	19179	151542	.0195
92	127039	30806	15403	111636	.0144
93	91973	24068	12034	79939	.0103
94	64853	17841	8920	55932	.0072
95	44772	13259	6629	38142	.0049
96	29852	9471	4735	25116	.0032
97	19213	6412	3206	16007	.0021
98	12141	4226	2113	10028	.0013
99	7482	2719	1359	6122	.0008
100	4491	1749	874	3616	.0005
101	2563	1066	533	2030	.0003
102	1389	596	298	1091	.0001
103	733	335	167	566	.0001
104	368	176	88	280	.0000
105	179	92	46	133	-
106	73	39	19	54	-
107	31	21	10	20	-
108	9	5	2	6	-
109	4	3	1	2	-
110	1	-	-	1	-
111	1	1	-	-	-
Total	8305904	1089746	554865	7761028	1.0
80-84				4931336	.6360
85-89				2126535	.2743
90-94				599943	.0774
95-99				95415	.0123
Total				7753229	1.0